QUICK
and Healthy
KETO ZONE
COOKBOOK

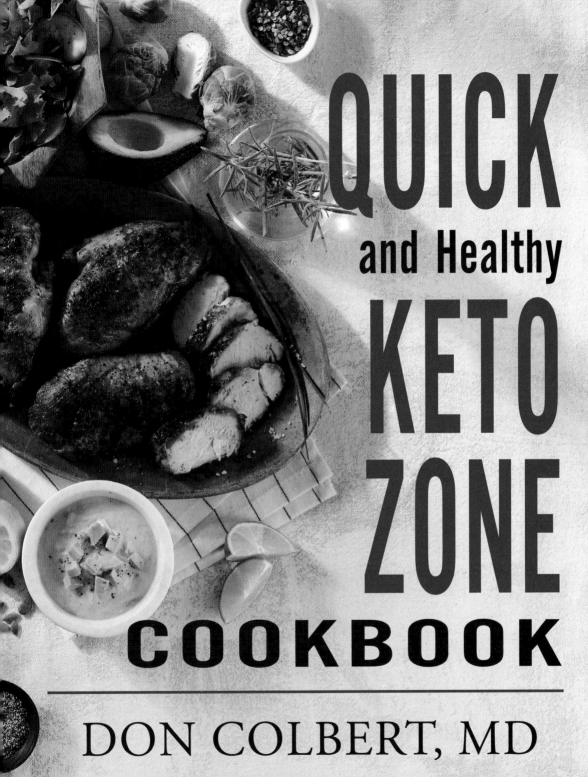

QUICK
and Healthy
KETO
ZONE
COOKBOOK

DON COLBERT, MD

WORTHY®
PUBLISHING

Worthy
Hachette Book Group
1290 Avenue of the Americas, New York, NY 10104

worthypublishing.com
twitter.com/worthypub

Worthy is a division of Hachette Book Group, Inc. The Worthy name and logo are trademarks of Hachette Book Group, Inc.

The publisher is not responsible for websites (or their content) that are not owned by the publisher.

Because each individual is different and has particular dietary needs or restrictions, the dieting and nutritional information provided in this book does not constitute professional advice and is not a substitute for expert medical advice. Individuals should always check with a doctor before undertaking a dieting, weight loss, or exercise regimen and should continue only under a doctor's supervision. When a doctor's advice to a particular individual conflicts with advice provided in this book, that individual should always follow the doctor's advice.

Calorie/Nutrient Analysis Notice: Though we strive to provide complete and accurate nutritional information, please note that there may be differences between the nutritional values we disclose and actual nutritional content of the food you prepare or eat. These variations can be the result of variations in ingredients or other variations in preparation, portion size, substitutions, etc.

Cover design by Marc Whitaker, MTW Design. Recipe development by Tammy Algood. Food styling by Teresa Blackburn. Food photography by Mark Boughton Photography. Managing editor: Leeanna Nelson
Print book interior design by Bart Dawson

Cataloging-in-Publication Data is on file with the Library of Congress.

ISBN: 978-1-68397-301-0

Printed in the United States of America

18 19 20 21 22 LBM 8 7 6 5 4 3 2 1

CONTENTS

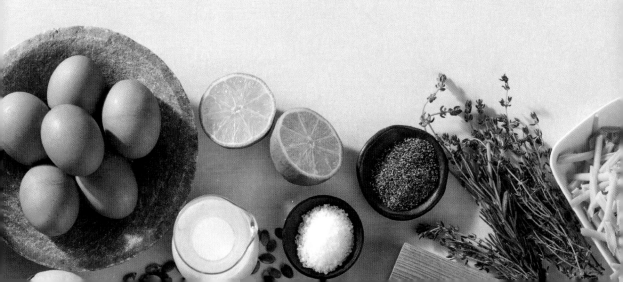

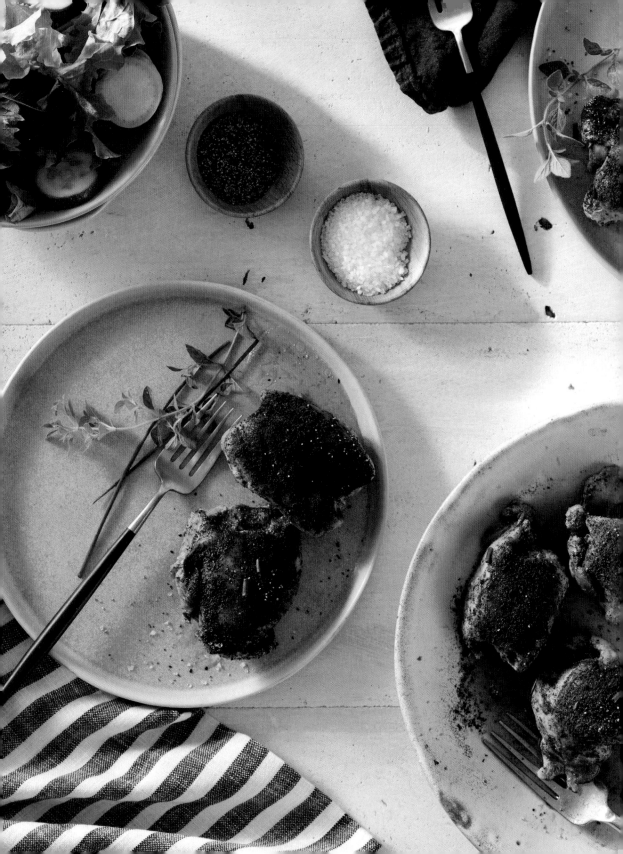

INTRODUCTION

For years I have treated patients who suffered from advanced cancers, obesity, type 2 diabetes, heart disease, mental illness, dementia, and much more. They needed help yesterday so they could be on the road to healing today. They were desperate, and they had no time to wait!

The answer was not a pill, medication, pharmaceutical drug, or surgery. The answer was a nutritional one completely based on the food we eat.

In a nutshell, this diet is low-carb, high-fat, and moderate protein. It is incredibly healthy, and not only does it work to cure or manage disease, it is, in my opinion, the best weight-loss method in the world.

I call it the Keto Zone diet.

Wait a minute, you might be thinking. *Did you just say this was a high-fat diet? How can fat be healthy?*

To clarify, the Keto Zone diet is a purposeful combination of reduced carbs, increased healthy fats, and a moderate amount of healthy proteins. Yes, it is high-fat, but it is also (and very importantly) low-carb and moderate-protein. These elements go together to create a body that is satisfied, alert, happy, and fat-burning.

When it comes to fats, not all are bad for you. However, we have been taught for so long that fats are bad that we have a very real and tangible fear of fat. And why not? The message from most doctors, food guidelines, trends magazines, and every other "authority" in life tells us in big, bold letters that fat is BAD.

In truth, healthy fats are good. They are necessary. They will help you lose weight. And no, they will not make you fat, clog your arteries, or cause you to drop dead.

The Keto Zone diet works. It also cures or manages countless diseases.

If you are ready for that, then come on! I suggest picking up a copy of *Dr. Colbert's Keto Zone Diet* to go along with this cookbook.

—Don Colbert, MD

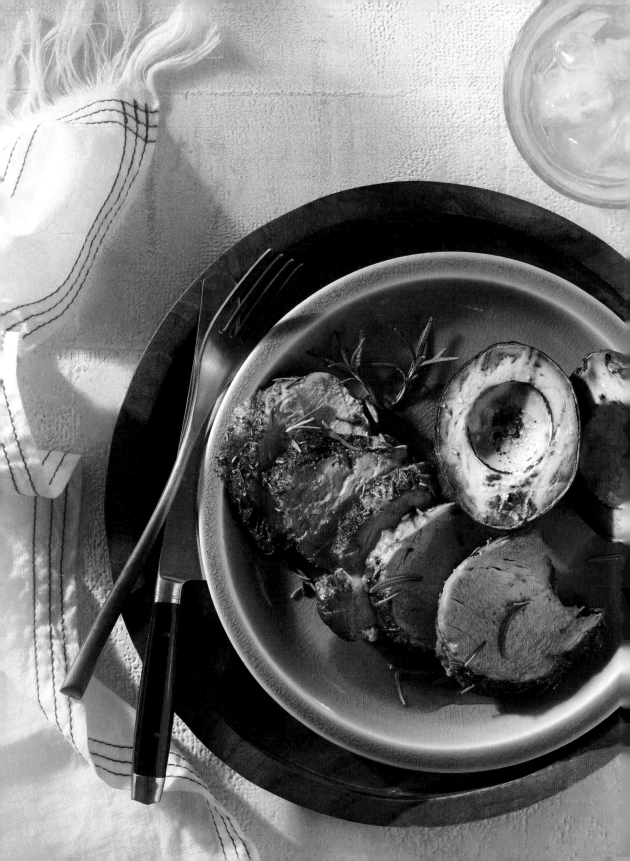

Part One
OVERVIEW OF
THE KETO ZONE DIET

My wife, Mary, is my greatest fan as well as my toughest critic. She is always honest and tells it like it is. I knew if she could do the Keto Zone diet, then anyone could.

Within roughly three months, she had lost about twenty pounds, eventually reaching her goal of thirty-five pounds of weight loss, and she has kept it off!

"I had no hunger cravings, no sugar or carb cravings, and no light-headedness. Quite honestly, it was far easier than I expected," she said.

Like most people, Mary lost four to five pounds the first week, most of which was water that the body naturally stores. After the first week, she lost one to two pounds of fat a week. We added in some exercise (brisk walking, thirty minutes a day, five days a week) to her routine, and she increased the fat-burning rate to two to three pounds a week. Even if you only lost a single pound per week, in a year that would be fifty-two pounds. Nobody would object to that! What is more, that type of gradual weight loss shows the person is on track and is staying in the Keto Zone, which is peak fat-burning mode.

"In addition to always being hungry, most people on a diet are not sure what they can and cannot eat, so I had Don tell me what to eat, how to shop, and how to do this in the real world," Mary explained.

We worked together to clear out our pantry of foods that would bump us out of the Keto Zone. All the processed foods in boxes were the first to go. We then bought the right ingredients and began to cook differently. Living in the Keto Zone was easier than she first expected.

Not long ago while we were traveling, Mary took pictures of food in restaurants that she could eat and still remain in the Keto Zone. It helped prove the point that if you want to stay in the zone, you can do it, even if you are eating out.

The Keto Zone diet is a unique program. You lose weight without starving yourself to death. But that is not all. On the Keto Zone diet, you can expect the following, usually:

- Virtually no hunger cravings
- Full appetite control
- A loss of 1 to 3 pounds per week
- Feelings of happiness
- Significant weight loss
- Plenty of energy
- Improved memory
- No brain fog
- Loss of belly fat
- No complaints there!

GETTING YOUR LIFE BACK

As I prescribed the Keto Zone diet to more and more patients, I could not help but want to share the tremendous health benefits of this diet. People are losing weight, especially belly fat, which is the most inflammatory fat in our bodies, but it was much more than weight loss. As the years went by, the list of ailments, diseases, symptoms, and health markers positively affected by the ketogenic diet continued to grow. Here is what I found with most of my patients:

- Sleep disorders usually improved
- Migraines usually improved
- Type 2 diabetes usually improved or was reversed
- ADHD and ADD usually improved
- Metabolic function usually restored
- Blood pressure usually lowered
- Fatty liver usually cured
- Irritable bowel syndrome (IBS) usually improved
- Dementia (mild to moderate) usually improved and, for some, cleared up
- Parkinson's (mild to moderate) usually improved and, for some, cleared up
- Chronic fatigue usually improved

- Energy levels significantly increased for many
- Mental illness, including schizophrenia and bipolar disorder, usually improved
- Fibromyalgia usually improved or cleared up
- Acne many times cleared up or improved
- Autoimmune diseases usually improved or occasionally were sent into remission
- Arthritis (mild, moderate, and even severe) usually improved or was managed, and, for some, completely cleared up
- Heartburn usually gone or improved
- Enlarged prostate usually improved or reduced to normal
- Gout usually cured, managed, or improved
- Small gallstones usually cleared up or improved
- Erectile dysfunction (ED) usually improved and sometimes resolved
- Immune system strengthened
- Aging process slowed down
- Joint aches usually improved or eliminated
- Hormones usually balanced or improved
- Polycystic ovary syndrome usually improved or was able to be managed

One more thing I noticed with my patients: they had tremendous hope! That alone was worth every effort to push them closer toward a healthy lifestyle.

I believe the Keto Zone diet is the healthiest diet in the world. The diet, in my opinion, is more important than any medicine, exercise, or supplements. The food that is in the diet is what makes it work. Nothing else compares for weight loss, for overcoming or managing sicknesses and disease, and for creating a healthy and balanced lifestyle going forward.

Redefining Healthy Foods

There are three foundational health truths that each one of us needs to understand in today's culture. Armed with that reality, we can navigate through life and achieve the results we want with greater ease.

We need to do things differently.

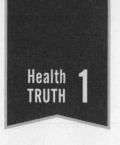
SEE SUGAR AND EXCESSIVE CARBOHYDRATES AS THE ENEMY

Recognize that we are not just talking about table sugar or candy. The excess carbohydrates and starches we eat are eventually broken down to sugar. Carbs also come in the forms of fruits, bread, certain vegetables (especially potatoes), pasta, beverages, sauces, condiments, most dairy products, canned goods, desserts, yogurt, cereals, grains (wheat, corn, rice, oats), juices, and much more.

Yes, exactly; sugar is in virtually everything we eat.

Carbohydrates in the form of wheat, corn, rice, and potatoes are the most consumed sources of carbs. Our bodies convert these carbs and starches to sugar, which spikes insulin levels, and elevated insulin levels cause one to store fat. Sweets and carbs invite disease in and are the main enemies of weight loss. Once excess sugar and carbs (in its various forms, such as breads, pasta, juice, and cereal) enter our bodies, they program one to store fat, especially belly fat.

If you are wondering if we are doomed to a life of bland food, know that we are not.

Or maybe we are doomed to a life of sickness? No to that as well.

As for sugars and sweeteners for beverages and cooking, there are several forms of natural sweeteners that are safe. I recommend stevia, monk fruit, and sweet alcohols such as erythritol and xylitol. These are healthy and have a low calorie count, which make them ideal for healthy living and weight loss in the Keto Zone diet. Stevia and monk fruit are both in powder and liquid forms, though liquid is a bit better. (Be careful not to use excessive amounts of xylitol since it can cause gastrointestinal disturbances.)

What about regular sugar, candy, syrup, honey, agave, juices, cookies, breads, pasta, pies, cakes, and all the other countless forms of "sweets" that we grew up on and do not want to leave behind? The answer is to avoid them for now and start making healthy desserts that help push you toward your weight-loss goals.

Health TRUTH 2

KNOW THAT ALL FAT IS NOT YOUR ENEMY

I used to think that saturated fat was bad. Come on, everybody has been taught that, right? But is it true? Consider this:

Once you understand and start eating healthy fats, you will control appetite, tame hunger, lose weight, eliminate inflammation, and find your body will usually start to heal itself.

That is a fact. And that is healthy. It is also a bit of a mental jump!

To start with, know that we are talking about choosing the right combination of fish oil, healthy monounsaturated fats, and limited amounts of healthy saturated fats (about 25% of your fat intake); minimizing polyunsaturated fats and choosing healthy ones (for example, walnuts, other tree nuts, seeds, and nut and seed butters); and never cooking with polyunsaturated fats. Also avoid deep fried foods and trans fats.

Admittedly, it may take awhile for the new reality—that certain fats are indeed good for you—to sink in and even longer for that reality to become a natural part of life.

Yes, it goes against much of what we have been taught, but it is impossible to argue that our current recommended low-fat, high-carb diet we have followed for generations is actually making us healthier. Quite the opposite is true!

How does eating healthy fats play a part in the Keto Zone diet? And how does it help you lose weight? In a nutshell, this is what happens when your body is in the Keto Zone:

Your body burns stored excess fat as fuel when you reduce your carb intake enough. The healthy fats aid in the fat burning, increased metabolism, appetite control, reduced food cravings, increased energy, feelings of happiness, and clear thinking.

Eating a moderate amount of protein along with the healthy fats and reduced carbohydrates turns your body into a fat-burning machine. It is not only natural and healthy; it is really incredible to experience.

For now, know that fat is not your enemy.

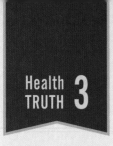

ACCEPT THAT THE RULES HAVE CHANGED

The third foundational health truth is for many the biggest "ah-ha" moment in their understanding of what the Keto Zone diet is, because it helps them understand how it works. When they understand this, all the other pieces of the puzzle seem to fall into place. That is because the rules have changed.

To set the stage, consider this question you may have asked yourself: *Why can't I eat what I used to and get away with it?*

My patients ask me this all the time. They are shocked and genuinely angry that their bodies cannot keep up with the foods and drinks they are used to consuming. All was fine back when they were younger, so where did these muffin tops, love handles, potbellies, menopots, and more come from?

What my patients have done is come face-to-face with the cold, hard, unyielding reality of carbohydrate sensitivity. This is their new norm, whether they like it or not.

Most people slowly build up a sensitivity to carbohydrates and become insulin resistant as they age, with the tipping point usually being around the age of fifty.

This carbohydrate sensitivity and insulin resistance are what translate directly into belly fat.

The great news is that carbohydrate sensitivity and insulin resistance can be broken down. For those seemingly stuck in a lose-lose battle with their weight, there is a way out. It is possible to get your body back on track, control your hormones, manage your appetite, and lose weight.

That is why lowering insulin levels, which is what happens in the Keto Zone diet, is so absolutely necessary. By lowering insulin levels, you enable your body to keep losing weight, as much as you want. When you control your insulin levels, you are the one in control.

OVERVIEW OF THE KETO ZONE DIET

On the Keto Zone diet, you lower your daily carb intake to around 20 grams per day, boost your healthy fat intake, and maintain a moderate protein intake. That causes your body to shift to burning fat rather than using the usual sugar as fuel. You have just shifted into the Keto Zone or your fat-burning zone! You are now burning fat as your main fuel and not sugar.

Your insulin numbers come completely under your control at this point, and you can eventually lose as much weight as you want. Carb sensitivity is not an issue because you have temporarily lowered your carb intake below your body's carbohydrate threshold for weight gain, and insulin levels drop dramatically, programming you for weight loss.

When your body is in this fat-burning mode, you are technically in the state of ketosis. Often misunderstood, the word *ketosis* is admittedly very scary sounding, which is one of the reasons why ketogenic diets as a whole have received such negative press. Scary! Bad! Dangerous! Unsafe! Deadly! In truth, ketosis is the natural, safe condition where your body is burning fat rather than sugar as its primary fuel source. You actually come close to ketosis when you sleep. If you eat dinner around 6 p.m. and drink only water before eating breakfast at 6 a.m., your body is very close to a ketosis state after twelve hours of fasting. Fasting longer than twelve hours does the same thing, even more so.

But after you eat breakfast or break your fast, your body usually does not return to ketosis again all day. That is because your body is busy digesting the food you have eaten and breaking down carbs and starches into sugar. If what you ate is the normal low-fat, high-carb diet, burning sugar is all that your body can do for the rest of the day.

Imagine instead if your body was burning fat all day long! Even better, imagine feeling full and satisfied, sharp and alert, with boundless energy and no food cravings for the entire day!

That is what typically happens to your body when you are in the Keto Zone.

That is how it works. That is the Keto Zone diet in a nutshell. It sounds so simple, and it really is.

Stay Full and in the Keto Zone

Food is the focus, so it is only normal to wonder exactly what the expectations and limits are for the Keto Zone diet. From the perspective of carbs, fats, and protein, here is an approximate framework of what you will eat while in the Keto Zone:

Carbs: 10 to 15 percent of daily caloric intake from healthy carbs, such as salad veggies, non-starchy vegetables, spices, and herbs.

Fats: 70 percent of daily caloric intake from healthy fats including omega-3 fats (fish oil), healthy monounsaturated fats, limited healthy saturated fats, and minimal healthy polyunsaturated fats.

Proteins: 10 to 15 percent of daily caloric intake from healthy protein, such as pasture-raised (or pastured) eggs and chicken, wild low-mercury fish, and grass-fed meats, aiming for around 1 gram of protein per 1 kilogram of weight.

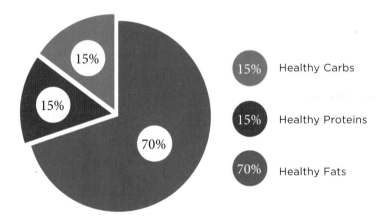

When you fuel your body with 10 to 15 percent healthy carbs, 70 percent healthy fats, and 10 to 15 percent healthy proteins, you are going to be in the peak metabolic fat-burning zone! It usually takes people one to three days to reach the Keto Zone (maybe seven to fourteen days for pre-diabetics and type 2 diabetics), but if it takes you longer than three days, rest assured you will get there.

These percentages are flexible in that if you need to increase fats a bit more or decrease proteins, or even eat more green veggies, you will usually remain in the Keto Zone. However, the 20 grams of carbs usually should not be increased until your desired weight is achieved.

You must be wondering, *how much fat is 70 percent of your diet?* We are only talking about approximately 8 to 10 tablespoons of fat per day for men, 6 to 8 tablespoons a day for women, and sometimes more. With the menus and recipes in the following chapters, this will be incredibly easy to accomplish. And you will usually feel full all day and all night as a result, while losing weight.

When you are in ketosis, your body naturally produces acids in the blood called *ketones*, which are flushed out in the urine. These trace amounts of ketones are a sign that your body is breaking down fat. It usually takes a few days for your body to get into the Keto Zone, and with the small amounts of ketones in your urine, the initial and easiest way to measure is with a urine test strip. These ketone strips, such as Ketostix, are inexpensive and readily available at a local pharmacy or health food store. (You can even cut the strips in half to save a few dollars.) See Appendix A for a source. To see if you are in ketosis, pass the ketone strip through your urine stream, then wait fifteen seconds and compare the strip to the color chart on the side of the bottle.

KCL: Keto Carb Limit

For health and life, you need certain proteins and fats, but your body does not technically need any carbohydrates (or sugars or starches). Our normal low-fat, high-carb diet provides us with too much of what we do not actually need. With starches and carbs as the base of the food pyramid, what do you expect, right? The average person clocks in around 200 to 300 grams of carbs a day.

Everyone has a specific ideal carb management number. Quite simply, eating more carbohydrates than that number equals weight gain; eating less equals weight loss.

I call this ideal carb management number your KCL, or Keto Carb Limit. Your KCL may be 20 grams or 50 grams or 75 grams or 100 grams per day. Nobody knows, but you will find your KCL as you put the Keto Zone diet to work in your life.

Finding your KCL is vitally important to your long-term weight loss and long-term health. For now, though, it is pretty safe to assume your KCL is usually somewhere between 20 and 100 grams per day. Once you have burned off the fat and reached your desired weight, you will usually have a new KCL number. Maybe it will be 50 grams or 75 grams or 100 grams or some other number. It will usually be higher than the fat-burning 20 grams. Finding your KCL (Keto Carb Limit) draws the line in the sand for weight loss and ideal health. If you reduce your carb intake below your ideal KCL, you will lose weight. It is inevitable.

Imagine losing weight and not being hungry. Most often, that is precisely what happens on the Keto Zone diet. Your hunger is usually controlled because your ghrelin and leptin levels eventually are under control. The most important hormone balance we need in our bodies for appetite control is the balance of leptin and ghrelin, and when those two hormones are balanced, we usually have appetite control!

The longer you stay in the Keto Zone, the easier it becomes and the more control you have over your appetite hormones. Appetite hormones may kick and scream, but eventually they will obey you and come into balance. They have no choice because they only have as much power as you give them, and food is power.

THE POWER OF FAT

The high-fat part of the Keto Zone diet (in the form of oils, butters, meats, nuts, and fish) accomplishes two main goals:

1. *To satisfy you:* These foods and especially the fats make you feel full, satisfied, without cravings or hunger, and happy for many hours.
2. *To nourish you:* These foods provide your body with the essential fatty acids, fat-soluble vitamins, and healthy fats in the correct ratios that will decrease inflammation in the body. (According to the 2005 Dietary Guidelines of America, a low intake of fats, less than 20 percent of calories, increases the risk of not getting enough vitamin E and essential fats.)

We need a balance of fats in our body. That is partly why a low-fat diet is inherently unhealthy. Deprive your body and brain of fats, especially your brain, and you will eventually have a host of problems. After all, your brain is about 60 percent fat, and a significant portion of the brain is composed of cholesterol, omega-3 fats, and phospholipids. The truth remains that your body needs certain fats—not every fat, nor in large quantities, but the right fats (that are healthy) and in the right amount. That is partly what makes the Keto Zone diet so unique and powerful.

The diet is also flexible in that if you find yourself still hungry, you can increase your fat intake a bit. This is vital for the Keto Zone diet because:

The only reason people fall out of the Keto Zone is because they're not eating enough fats or they are eating too much protein or too many carbs.

If you need to increase your fats especially monounsaturated fats and, for some, saturated fats, that is fine. It is not going to hurt you because you have decreased your sugar and carb intake so much that excessive oxidation, inflammation, or insulin spikes will not occur. For cholesterol concerns refer to Appendix D in *Dr. Colbert's Keto Zone Diet*. If you have high cholesterol, use avocado oil instead of butter called for in these recipes.

THE POWER OF PROTEIN

Protein is a must for your body. Specifically, you need nine essential amino acids (histidine, isoleucine, leucine, lysine, methionine, phenylalanine, threonine, tryptophan, and valine), and the only way to get them is through the food you eat.

The Keto Zone diet limits protein intake because if you eat too much of it, all fat burning usually stops. It is not a matter of healthy proteins or carbohydrates. Rather, it is the fact that too much protein may bump you out of the Keto Zone.

The ideal protein intake ratio for the Keto Zone diet is approximately 1 gram of protein per 1 kilogram (2.2 pounds) of body weight.

That breaks down to be about 20 to 30 grams of protein per meal, with 60 to 140 grams as the maximum amount for a day. So someone weighing 180 pounds needs about 80 grams of protein a day, or 27 grams per meal. At 125, 150, or 250 pounds, that is 19, 23, or 38 grams respectively per meal.

The fact that the Keto Zone diet is moderate-protein is part of what makes it unique among other ketogenic diets. Not only does protein intake need to be low enough to avoid gluconeogenesis (where your body turns excess proteins into sugar), it also needs to be high enough to provide your body with the essential amino acids that it needs.

This is a delicate balance, one that the Keto Zone diet is able to provide for your body.

In addition, the Keto Zone diet goes a step further with healthy sources of protein and healthy sources of fat from plants and pastured or grass-fed animals. This is ideal for fat burning as well as ideal for long-term health. I do not recom-mend processed meats such as bacon, sausage, ham, etc. on a regular basis since they increase your risk of certain cancers.

THE POWER OF CARBS

As we have discussed, the primary goal of the Keto Zone diet is to reduce your daily carbohydrate intake to below your body's carbohydrate threshold for weight gain. This in turn causes your body to burn excess fats rather than sugar as its fuel source, and your body begins to burn your stored fat as fuel.

The sugar your body usually burns is glucose, which is produced from the carbs (breads, sugar, pasta, potatoes, juices, sodas, fruits, and sugary beverages) you eat or drink. Any extra glucose is either stored in your liver or muscles as glycogen or converted to fat.

By lowering your carb intake, your insulin levels also drop, and your metabolism eventually shifts into fat-burning mode. Eating foods that are Keto Zone-healthy speeds up the fat-burning process (in the form of a high amount of healthy fats and a moderate amount of healthy protein), which helps you control your appetite and reach your goal weight.

Of course, not every carb, starch, or sugar is created equal. By its nature, everything you eat has a value or number associated with it. For example, 12 ounces of green leafy vegetables have a lower carb value (glycemic index) than 12 ounces of potatoes, and 12 ounces of bread have a different carb value than 12 ounces of broccoli.

Net carbs is a number achieved by subtracting fiber carbs from total carbs. A few nuts, for example, may have a total of 10 carbs, but with 5 fiber carbs, the net carb value is going to be 5. Knowing the net carbs of food can help you choose the best carbs for losing weight.

The limit of 20 grams of carbs is the net carb number. Green veggies are the best source for getting in your needed fiber while staying within the carb limit on the Keto Zone diet.

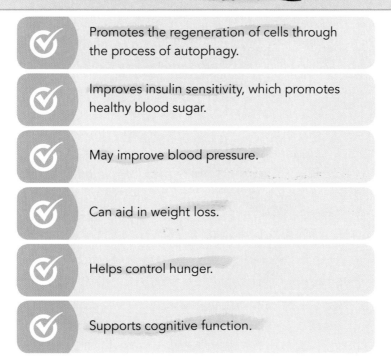

THE BENEFITS OF INTERMITTENT FASTING

Not eating from 6 PM or after dinner until 10 AM or about 16 hours. Start intermittent fasting ~~one day a week~~.

✓ Promotes the regeneration of cells through the process of autophagy.

✓ Improves insulin sensitivity, which promotes healthy blood sugar.

✓ May improve blood pressure.

✓ Can aid in weight loss.

✓ Helps control hunger.

✓ Supports cognitive function.

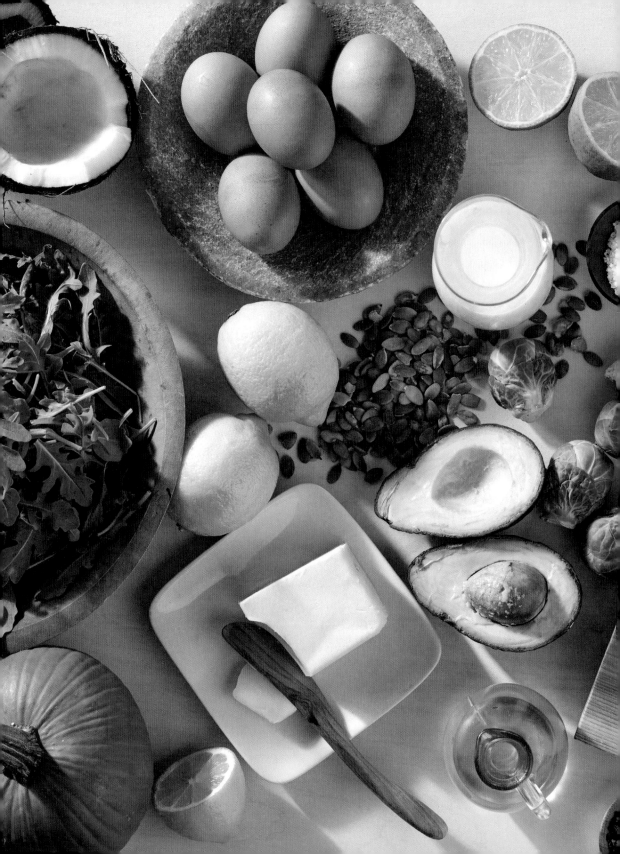

Part Two
THE KETO ZONE DIET
IN ACTION

You already know how and why the Keto Zone diet is the healthiest, fastest, safest, and easiest way to lose weight. Now it is time to put that knowledge into action.

The best place to begin is with the big picture of what it takes to implement the Keto Zone diet. It looks like this:

1. Know where you are aiming.
2. Go shopping for the right ingredients.
3. Get in the Keto Zone.
4. Stay in the Keto Zone with the right menu plans.
5. Discover your KCL number to maintain your ideal weight.

It is always wise and healthy to keep your reasons for going on the Keto Zone diet handy. Some patients have told me, "I'm going to get on the Keto Zone diet, lose weight, and then get on it later for detox or to lose weight again if I need to."

That is great. Using the Keto Zone as a detox program, weight-loss program, or both makes great sense. Some want specifically to improve or reverse their type 2 diabetes. Others want to prevent neurological disease, cancer, heart disease, or autoimmune diseases. On the general health level, some people are pleased to find out that being on a ketogenic diet means they are much less susceptible to viruses and bacterial infections. For me, I remember my father and am thankful that ketogenic diets have great potential to both prevent and sometimes reverse Alzheimer's.

For you, your motivating "why" may be specifically weight loss, health-related, or even future-focused. Whatever it is that moves you to take action, keep it fresh and in front of you as you dive into the amazing Keto Zone diet.

GETTING IN THE KETO ZONE

How fast can I get into the Keto Zone?

The short answer: it depends on your body.

Usually, it takes two to five days to get into the Keto Zone and begin to produce minor amounts of ketones (0.5–5 millimolar on the urine test strips) that show your body is in the fat-burning mode. It may take your body as long as one to two weeks. Some of my patients who are very carbohydrate sensitive and insulin resistant, or who have pre-diabetes, type 2 diabetes, or are very overweight, have taken almost three weeks to get into the Keto Zone. Rarely, some people need to lower their carb intake to only 10 grams of carbs a day to enter the Keto Zone.

For most people, however, the Keto Zone becomes a reality around day two to five, but rest assured, your body will eventually enter the Keto Zone. Keep eating the foods that get you into the Keto Zone, and eventually you will find yourself right in the center of the Keto Zone. It will happen. Trust me. It is inevitable.

Commonly, people will notice their ketone levels in trace ketones as they enter the Keto Zone around day two or day three, and by day five they are usually deep into the Keto Zone. You will get there, I promise. And though it is a great feeling when you do reach the Keto Zone, it is far more satisfying and fun when you see the fat melting away.

As for falling out of the Keto Zone, that can only happen if you do not eat enough fats, eat too much protein, or eat too many carbs. Just keep an eye on your ketone levels and adjust your foods accordingly, but if you stick with the diet, you will stay in the Keto Zone. Worst case, if you happen to fall out of the Keto Zone for one reason or another, whether by accident or on purpose, do not berate yourself or feel bad about it. You are usually only two or three Keto Zone meals (twelve hours) away from reentering the Keto Zone. Remember, after you fast for about twelve hours overnight, typically you'll be in mild ketosis. Another option is to take Instant Ketones, which allow you to get back into the Keto Zone usually within an hour. (See Appendix A.)

The good news is you can stay in the Keto Zone and keep burning fat for as long as you want.

CLEANING HOUSE

On clean-out day, here are some of the things that need to go:

- *Boxed food:* Get rid of packaged processed foods in a bag or box. They contain too many carbs, sugars, artificial sweeteners, hydrogenated oils, or refined oils to keep you in the Keto Zone. That means no pasta, breads, bagels, pretzels, chips, cereals, cookies, or frozen desserts.
- *Wheat, grains, beans:* Get rid of all flour, grains, rye, oats, corn, wheat, popcorn, barley, rice, brown rice, beans, peas, hummus, and lentils whether dried or in cans.
- *Unhealthy oils and fats:* Margarine, soy, and oils (sunflower, cottonseed, canola, soybean, corn, grape-seed, rapeseed, or safflower) need to go.
- *Canned goods:* Foods in metal cans, especially canned veggies, are notorious for containing BPA (bisphenol A), which disrupts our hormones. By imitating estrogen, it can fool the body into thinking that it is estrogen. In research, animals exposed to low levels of BPA had higher rates of diabetes, breast and prostate cancers, reproductive problems, low sperm count, obesity, and other negative effects. Not all canned food contains BPA, but they do contain unhealthy additives (to extend shelf life) and sugary juices (with many fruits and veggies) that can bump you out of the Keto Zone.
- *Sugar and artificial sweeteners:* Get rid of them all. Artificial sweeteners are unhealthy and mess with your appetite hormones. Regular sugar, syrups, honey, and agave should be removed, or put away if it is not too tempting. For now, use stevia or monk fruit (also called lohan guo) powder or liquid or sweet alcohols (erythritol and xylitol) because these are healthy and low carb.
- *Dairy:* Other than hard cheeses, heavy whipping cream, cream cheese, and grass-fed butter, all other dairy products should go. It is best to choose organic grass-fed dairy products and to consume dairy only every three to four days.
- *Low-fat:* Foods labeled "low-fat" or "fat-free" are usually especially bad for you because of added sugar and almost always throw you out of the Keto Zone.

- *Sauces and condiments:* Most sauces and condiments, like ketchup, have added sugars, so avoid them entirely or read the label and use sparingly. Spices such as pepper, salt, onion, garlic, and herbs are fine and have very low to virtually no carbs.
- *Beverages:* Get rid of all sodas, sports drinks, smoothies, prepared and sweetened coffees and teas, and drinks with artificial sweeteners.
- *Fruit juices:* Fresh-squeezed orange juice, though delicious, is very high in sugar. It instantly will sabotage your diet and bump you out of the Keto Zone. Remove *all* fruit juices.
- *Alcohol:* It is just best to cut out all alcohol. It will mess with your daily carb intake limit and bump you out of the Keto Zone. It also gives you brain fog and food cravings, and it reduces your ability to resist cravings. For now, just remove it from your diet.
- *Fruit:* Fruit like bananas, grapes, mangos, oranges, peaches, pears, pineapples, and plums, though delicious and healthy, contain too much sugar for you to stay in the Keto Zone.
- *Dried fruit:* Dried fruit, though natural and healthy, are high in fructose. For now, cut them out.
- *Jams, jellies, and preserves:* These have way too much sugar.
- *Chocolate and candy:* Except for 85 percent or higher low-sugar dark chocolate or dark chocolate with stevia, no other chocolate or candy works with the Keto Zone diet.
- *Some vegetables need to go as well:* Carrots, potatoes, beets, sweet potatoes, yams, and winter squashes (like acorn and butternut) have to go, as they are starches.

RESTOCKING YOUR SHELVES

The intake of 70 percent fats, 15 percent proteins, and 15 percent carbs is the framework, but the actual ingredients you choose are up to you. Here is a good outline to begin with:

Proteins (15 Percent)

The ratio of protein you need per day is 1 gram of protein per 2.2 pounds you weigh.

308# : 140g/day = 46.6g/meal (6.6oz/meal)

250 pounds: 114 g. protein per day = 38 g. per meal (5 to 6 oz. protein)
180 pounds: 80 g. protein per day = 27 g. per meal (4 oz. protein)
150 pounds: 68 g. protein per day = 23 g. per meal (3 to 3.5 oz. protein)

Remember that 1 ounce of protein from eggs, fish, chicken, or steak is approximately 7 grams of protein. That makes the math pretty easy. Per meal, that is about 3 to 4 ounces of protein for women and 3 to 6 ounces of protein for men. How you choose to meet that need is up to you.

Fish (wild is best and low in mercury)

- Wild Salmon
- Halibut
- Anchovies
- Perch
- Pollock
- Sole
- Tilapia
- Trout
- Herring
- Sardines
- Tuna (tongol)
- Flounder

Shellfish (wild is best)

- Clams
- Scallops
- Oysters
- Shrimp
- Squid
- Crab

Poultry (pastured organic is best)

- Eggs
- Chicken
- Duck
- Goose
- Cornish Hen
- Quail
- Pheasant
- Turkey

Meat (grass-fed organic is best)

- Beef
- Goat
- Lamb
- Pork
- Veal
- Venison

Dairy (grass-fed organic is best)

Remember, even though dairy and nuts are listed under protein, they include carbs that count toward your 20 grams per day limit. The carb numbers here are net carbs (total carbs – fiber = net carbs).

- Grass-fed butter: 2 Tbsp., 1 g. net carb
- Organic cheese: 4 oz. per day maximum, 1 g. net carb per ounce
- Organic cream cheese: 2 Tbsp., 0.8 g. net carb
- Organic full cream (heavy whipping cream), 0 g. net carb

Nuts

- Almond milk: 1 cup, 1 g. net carb
- Coconut milk: 1 cup, 1 g. net carb
- Almonds: 24 nuts (1 oz.), 2.3 g. net carbs
- Almond butter: 1 Tbsp., 2.5 g. net carbs
- Cashews: 18 nuts (1 oz.), 7.7 g. net carbs
- Peanuts: 35 nuts (1 oz.), 2.2 g. net carbs
- Peanut butter: 1 Tbsp., 2.4 g. net carbs (avoid most processed peanut butter since they usually contain hydrogenated fats)
- Pecans: 10 whole (1 oz.), 4 g. net carbs
- Macadamias: 8 medium-sized nuts (1 oz.), 4 g. net carbs
- Hazelnuts: 12 nuts (1 oz.), 2.3 g. net carbs
- Walnuts: 10 whole (1 oz.), 3 g. net carbs
- Coconut, fresh shredded: ½ cup, 6 g. net carbs
- Coconut, unsweetened dried: 1 oz., 7 g. net carbs
- Coconut cream butter: 2 Tbsp., 2 g. net carbs

Raw whole nuts are best, but roasted is fine. Note that some nuts, such as cashews, are higher in carbs. Excessive intake of nuts or consuming higher-carb nuts such as cashews (and peanuts, even though it is a legume) can throw you out of the Keto Zone and may rarely trigger flu-like symptoms for some. If nuts cause flu-like symptoms, then stop eating them or use them sparingly.

Carbs (15 Percent)

Basically, think salad vegetables and vegetables that you would cook. Salads are measured in cups (1 cup), while cooked vegetables are measured in half cups (½ cup).

Roughly speaking, you are going to eat about 2 to 6 cups of salad and 1 to 2 cups of cooked veggies per day, but you can usually eat as much as you want of green leafy veggies, and use generous amounts of extra-virgin olive oil (2 to 3 tablespoons) and apple cider vinegar in a ratio of three parts olive oil to one part apple cider vinegar. Here are many of the common vegetables you can enjoy. The carb numbers listed here are net carbs.

Raw Veggies (organic is best)

- Avocado: 3 slices (1 oz.), 2 g. net carbs; 2 Tbsp. mashed (1 oz.), 2 g. net carbs
- Broccoli pieces: 1 cup, 1.6 g. net carbs
- Green beans: 1 cup, 4.2 g. net carbs
- Cabbage: 1 cup, 2.2 g. net carbs
- Celery: 1 rib, 0.8 g. net carb
- Cucumber: 1 cup, 2 g. net carbs
- Mixed greens: 1 cup, 0.4 g. net carb
- Black olives: 5 count, 0.7 g. net carb
- Green olives: 5 count, 0 g. net carb
- Onion: 2 Tbsp., 1.5 g. net carbs
- Green pepper: 1 cup, 4.2 g. net carbs
- Romaine lettuce: 1 cup, 0.4 g. net carb
- Spinach: 1 cup, 0.2 g. net carb
- Tomato: 1 small (3 to 4 oz.), 2.5 g. net carbs

Cooked Veggies

- Green beans: ½ cup, 2.9 g. net carbs
- Bok choy: ½ cup, 0.2 g. net carb
- Broccoli: ½ cup, 1.7 g. net carbs
- Collard greens: ½ cup, 2 g. net carbs
- Eggplant: ½ cup, 2 g. net carbs
- Kale: ½ cup, 2.4 g. net carbs

- Brussels sprouts: ½ cup, 3.6 g. net carbs
- Cauliflower: ½ cup, 0.9 g. net carb
- Button mushrooms: ½ cup, 4.6 g. net carbs
- Onion: ½ cup, 8.6 g. net carbs
- Asparagus: ½ cup, 1.19 g. net carbs
- Spinach: ½ cup, 2.2 g. net carbs
- Green pepper: ½ cup, 3.8 g. net carbs
- Tomato: ½ cup, 8.6 g. net carbs
- Zucchini: ½ cup, 1.5 g. net carbs

Oils (70 Percent)

Oils have no carbs so they are ideal for food satisfaction, decreasing hunger and cravings, sticking to the 20 gram carb limit, and providing your body with the optimal fuel source.

Extra-virgin olive oil and avocado oil are ideal for salad dressings. You can cook with coconut oil, avocado oil, ghee, and grass-fed butter. These oils are also good for sautéing.

MCT oil is not only great for increasing energy, but it also pushes you into the Keto Zone. The fat from MCT oil is not stored; it only burns as fuel. I recommend it especially in your coffee in the mornings (1 to 2 tablespoons); I prefer the MCT oil powder for my coffee. Start with the lower amount of MCT to avoid loose stools. (See Appendix A).

These are ideal healthy oils (serving size with oils is 1 tablespoon) for the Keto Zone. You can also choose nut butters.

Saturated Fats (best for cooking)
- Grass-fed butter
- Extra-virgin coconut oil
- MCT oil (powder, liquid, or capsule)
- Ghee (clarified butter, grass-fed)
- Palm oil (sustainable only)
- Cocoa butter (usually not for cooking)

Monounsaturated Fats
- Extra-virgin olive oil
- Avocado oil
- Almond oil
- Macadamia nut oil

Miscellaneous

From spices to fruits to beverages, these foods, separate from fats, veggies, and proteins, are safe to eat on the Keto Zone diet. Be sure to include their carb count in your daily 20 gram limit.

Fruit

- Blueberries, fresh: ¼ cup, 4.1 g. net carbs
- Blueberries, frozen: ¼ cup, 3.7 g. net carbs
- Blackberries, fresh: ¼ cup, 2.7 g. net carbs
- Blackberries, frozen: ¼ cup, 4.1 g. net carbs
- Raspberries, fresh: ¼ cup, 1.5 g. net carbs
- Raspberries, frozen: ¼ cup, 1.8 g. net carbs
- Strawberries, fresh, sliced: ¼ cup, 1.8 g. net carbs
- Strawberries, frozen: ¼ cup, 2.6 g. net carbs
- Lemon juice: 2 Tbsp., 2.1 g. net carbs
- Lime juice: 2 Tbsp., 2.6 g. net carbs

Beverages

- Water
- Sparkling water
- Coffee
- Green tea
- Black tea
- Yerba mate
- Nut milks (almond and coconut have low sugar), nut milks are low-carb and good to use in smoothies. Just be sure to use the low-carb types with 1 gram or less of carbs per 8-ounce serving.

Supplements

- A comprehensive multivitamin with vitamin D (1000 to 2000 IU) and magnesium (400 mg) a day
- Omega-3 (EPA/DHA) 1 to 2 g. per day and/or krill oil (350 to 1000 mg) per day
- Electrolyte packets: in first month of the Keto Zone diet, people often need extra magnesium, sodium, and potassium

- A digestive enzyme with extra lipase to help with the digestion of fats, especially for those fifty-five and older

Spices and Condiments

- Garlic: 1 large clove, 0.9 g. net carb
- Ginger: 1 Tbsp., 0.8 g. net carb
- Pesto sauce: 1 Tbsp., 0.6 g. net carb
- Apple cider vinegar: 1 Tbsp., 1 g. net carbs
- Sea salt: 1 tsp., 0 g. net carb
- Himalayan salt (pink): 1 tsp., 0 g. net carb
- Rosemary: 1 tsp., 1 g. net carb
- Turmeric: 1 tsp., 1 g. net carb
- Oregano: 1 tsp., 1 g. net carb
- Thyme: 1 tsp., 1 g. net carb
- Black pepper: 1 tsp., 0.5 g. net carb
- Vanilla extract: 1 tsp., 0.5 g. net carb
- Cinnamon 1 tsp., 2 g. net carbs

EATING OUT AND STAYING IN THE KETO ZONE

You can eat out and stay in the Keto Zone. You may have to bring your own olive oil or avocado oil and apple cider vinegar or grass-fed butter (as I do), but it is certainly doable.

Whether you are traveling or just going out to eat, you can make it work and keep yourself in the Keto Zone.

Eating out is also a good way to treat yourself. For a long while, every Monday night Mary and I would go out to eat at a local restaurant and have a salad with mozzarella cheese, tomatoes, basil, olive oil, a little balsamic vinegar, and a lot of herbs and spices. It is called a Caprese salad. It was delicious, and we both stayed in the Keto Zone.

Whether it is breakfast, lunch, or dinner, get creative and make the restaurant's menu fit your Keto Zone diet.

If you happen to get bumped out of the Keto Zone, you may feel it the next day. That is fine. Just get back into it, and usually within a day you will be back in the groove. You can also take the Instant Ketones found in Appendix A and you'll usually be back in the Keto Zone within an hour.

TROUBLESHOOTING IF NEEDED

Over the years in working with patients who are ready to jump into the Keto Zone to lose weight or combat a sickness, a lot of questions naturally arise. Every question is a good one, but here are many that I have received. I hope they will be the questions you wanted to ask.

Why start with the extreme 20 grams carb limit?

The 20 grams of carbs per day is a limit that will usually be low enough to kick-start healthy nutritional ketosis where the body burns fat for fuel rather than burning sugars. Most people hover around 50 to 75 grams as their ideal KCL (Keto Carb Limit) number, which means 20 grams is low enough to start the fat-burning engines. If we started at 50 grams of carbs and your KCL is 50 grams of carbs, you would neither gain nor lose weight. This is precisely the point you want to reach eventually, but only after you have achieved your ideal weight.

How long can I stay in the Keto Zone?

Stay as long as you want. When you reach your ideal weight, increase your carb intake little by little until you see you are dropping in and out of ketosis. This is your KCL number. Staying at your KCL number usually means no more weight gain.

How can I max this out?

If you want to shed as much fat as possible, you can lower protein intake to 5 to 10 percent of total calories, boost fats to 80 percent, and lower carbs to 10 percent healthy green veggies. Add twenty to thirty minutes of high-intensity interval training (bike, treadmill, elliptical, or weight lifting) three to five times a week, and you may be burning one pound of fat each day, especially if you drink Keto Zone coffee instead of eating breakfast. (If you are over forty-five years of age, getting a stress test or EKG before starting high-intensity training would be wise.) If you have not been on a regular exercise program, do not start with high-intensity interval training.

If you want to lose one pound a day, skip breakfast and drink a cup or two of Keto Zone coffee, which is organic, single-sourced coffee with 1 to 2 tablespoons of MCT oil powder or MCT oil. (You can add stevia or ½ teaspoon of dark cocoa to taste.) It will put you in the Keto Zone, and you will usually not be hungry for three to five hours or longer. Then have a Keto Zone lunch and dinner, and you'll have jump-started your metabolism. I prefer MCT oil powder over MCT oil because too much MCT oil may cause diarrhea, whereas MCT oil powder usually will not. Once in the Keto Zone many people find they are completely satisfied with only two meals a day. This will also speed up weight loss and you will enjoy the health benefits of intermittent fasting.

What if I keep falling in and out of the Keto Zone?
It would seem that you need to adjust things slightly. My guess is that you are getting too many carbs, but it may also be too much protein or not enough fats. First, look at your carbs and then your proteins. It would not hurt to increase your fat intake slightly and make sure it's a 25-50/50-75 mix of saturated and monounsaturated fats. See Appendix D of *Dr. Colbert's Keto Zone Diet* for instructions on lowering cholesterol levels.

How do I check my ketone levels?
When you are in the Keto Zone, your ketones will usually register at 0.5 to 3 millimolars; however, 0.5 to 5 millimolars is also good. For the first month or two, use urine test strips to measure your ketone (acetoacetate) levels, but beyond that a ketone breath analyzer (to measure acetone) or a blood ketone monitor (to measure beta-hydroxybutyrate) will work best. Either can be found online, but I prefer the ketone breath analyzer, such as the one made by Ketonix.

Do I need to count my calories?
No, you should not have to count your calories. Just follow the recommended food options, and you usually will be fine. There are times when you will need to count carbs to make sure you are below the 20-gram threshold per day, but even that may not be required if you stay close to the recommended foods and portion sizes.

What if I get hungry during the day?
If you get hungry during the day, it usually means you are not getting enough fats. Increase your fats with grass-fed butter, healthy monounsaturated oils, nuts, or

cheese. (If you are hungry because you bumped yourself out of the Keto Zone, that could be the result of too much carbs or too much protein.) Watch the carbs!

Can I still eat dairy?

If you want dairy, go ahead and eat it, but it is best to alternate days or use small amounts, about 4 ounces a day. Use organic, grass-fed heavy whipping cream (best) or half-and-half, both of which are 1 gram of carbs per 2 tablespoons, in your coffee rather than milk. Overall, it is hard to stay in the Keto Zone and under 20 grams of carbs if you eat excessive amounts of dairy. It usually works best not to eat dairy every day but to alternate dairy every two to four days.

Can I still eat chocolate?

Absolutely! In fact, I recommend it. Dark (85 percent cacao) low-sugar choc-olate or dark chocolate with stevia instead of sugar a couple times a day boosts dopamine levels, which give you happy feelings, help turn off food cravings, and improve blood flow to the brain. Enjoy a couple of squares once or twice a day. I usually enjoy two small squares of dark chocolate every evening for my dessert.

Can I eat any bread at all?

Apart from a few specialty breads, such as seed bread, which boasts about 1 gram of carbs per slice, it is best to avoid all breads. For now, eliminate grains, breads, pasta, starches, potatoes, corn, rice, oats, and cereals. If you crave a hamburger or sandwich, use lettuce leaves instead of bread.

Do I have to eat three meals a day?

Some people will only want two meals a day. Some may even go down to a single meal a day, along with their Keto Zone coffee, but it is up to you. As long as you are getting your necessary fats and proteins and green veggie carbs and are staying in the Keto Zone, you can decide for yourself how often to eat. Typically, the more snacks you eat, the less weight you lose.

How much exercise is required?

Exercise helps you stay in the Keto Zone. It also speeds up your weight loss, boosts energy, burns fat, increases muscle, and revs up your metabolic rate, which means increased fat burning when you are resting. Technically, it takes a 3,500-calorie deficit to lose a pound of fat, so if you burn an extra 500 calories per day with exercise, in a week that is an extra pound of fat loss. A brisk walk twenty to thirty minutes a day, five times a week, is usually sufficient to accomplish this. By being in the Keto Zone, you will lose about one to two pounds a week anyway. Adding exercise usually increases that to one to two pounds of fat loss per week, especially high intensity exercise, such as interval training.

Is there a special way to cook all this healthy food?
Cooking over low heat is important. The higher the heat, the more denatured, oxidized, and damaged the food becomes, and that means fewer health benefits. Never cook with polyunsaturated fats (soybean oil, corn oil, grape-seed oil, etc.). The best cooking oil is ghee, grass-fed butter, avocado oil, or coconut oil. When you broil or grill, use lower heat, and do not burn or char the meat. Veggies are best steamed or sautéed. Bake at 320 degrees or less, use a slow cooker, and do not use a microwave to cook food. Eggs are healthiest when poached, soft boiled, or over easy. If you scramble your eggs, use low heat so you do not oxidize the yolk.

How much is all this going to cost me?
Fats are cheap, and with 70 percent of the diet being fats, it likely will be less expensive than you think. The protein, 10 to 15 percent of the diet, is the most expensive part, but we are not eating all that much protein. The remaining 15 percent is green veggies, also pretty cheap. All in all, the Keto Zone diet is very economical. It may even save you money.

What if I get diarrhea, bloating, or gas?
This will usually stop after a couple days as your body adjusts to the new high-fat diet. You can decrease magnesium a bit since it may trigger diarrhea in some people. Taking too much MCT oil or olive oil can also trigger diarrhea. Cut back your dose of these oils if diarrhea occurs, and when it stops, increase the dose slowly and gradually. People over age fifty-five may need a digestive enzyme containing extra lipase to help them digest fats better and to curb diarrhea.

What if I get constipated?

You need more water (1 to 2 quarts per day at least), fiber (from veggies or seeds), and magnesium (200 milligrams twice a day is normal, double if constipated). Increasing olive oil intake will also help.

What if I get light-headed, have brain fog, or feel sluggish?

You probably need sodium in the form of salted almonds or other salted nuts, a clear broth soup (like bouillon), or an electrolyte packet containing sodium, magnesium, and potassium. You may also need to increase your sea salt or Himalayan salt intake.

What if I have eye twitches, heart flutters, or muscle cramps?

You probably need more magnesium or potassium. A handful of nuts is high in magnesium. Or you can take 400 milligrams of chelated magnesium supplement. Half an avocado contains twice the potassium of a banana, and without the carbs. (A banana will bump you out of the Keto Zone.) Again, an electrolyte packet will help if it contains magnesium, potassium, and sodium, but no sugar.

What if I eat or drink something and then feel groggy?

That food or drink (for example, peanuts, coffee, cheese, whipping cream, etc.) may be causing inflammation. You could be sensitive to it, or it may contain mold toxins or other toxins, or perhaps what you ate was simply too high in carbs. Minimize it if you can, avoid it if you need to, and keep your carb intake at 20 grams or lower per day. Remember, if you've been in the Keto Zone for a while and then eat a lot of carbs, you may have symptoms of the keto flu, which I discuss in my book *Dr. Colbert's Keto Zone Diet*. Simply lower your carbs and take Instant Ketones (see Appendix A) and it usually pulls you right out of the fog and back into the Keto Zone.

What if I feel achy?

Again, the foods you are eating may be causing inflammation. Peanuts, foods high in mold toxins (such as moldy nuts and moldy berries), and dairy are common causes. Alternate dairy every three to four days or avoid altogether. There are other food and drink choices.

What if I urinate a lot more than normal?

When your body shifts into ketosis, insulin levels go down. The elevated insulin has caused you to retain water, so you will lose about four to five pounds of water weight your first week in the Keto Zone as your kidneys excrete the excess fluids. Drink sufficient water (usually 2 quarts a day for the first week and 1 to 2 quarts thereafter), along with taking sodium, potassium, and magnesium, during this time. The frequent urination will usually stop after the first week. Also, for the first week, you may need to urinate one to two times during the night.

What if I am not getting enough fiber?

Fiber is important, but you will usually get plenty with the veggies on the Keto Zone diet. You can add seeds (for example, chia seeds, sunflower seeds, psyllium seeds or husks, 1 to 2 tablespoon one to two times per day) in a few weeks, but seeds also have carbs. For now, the fiber in the green vegetables will usually be sufficient.

What if I eat too many carbs by accident?

You can usually be back in the Keto Zone within an hour if you take Instant Ketones (see Appendix A).

What if my gallbladder acts up?

Often women who have done a lot of low-fat diets and vegetarians may have gall-bladder issues without realizing it. Their gallbladder may contain sludge or may not be functioning properly since fats usually help the gallbladder function better. Healthy fats, such as 1 to 2 tablespoons of olive oil two to three times a day, will usually flush out the gallbladder.

Initially, you may need a teaspoon of olive oil every hour, for four to eight hours, to slowly get the gallbladder functioning normally again. Take it slow and in low amounts if you need to, and consult your doctor if the pain persists; you may have undiagnosed gallstones or sludge in your gallbladder.

What if my four pounds of water loss comes back?

When you first went into the Keto Zone, your body probably dumped about four pounds of stored water and glycogen. If you bump yourself out of the Keto Zone, it is possible that you may suddenly gain that water back from a single meal (by eating pizza or a baked potato, for example). Though it may seem scary, you know what happened. Stick to the Keto Zone diet, and you will lose those 4 pounds of water in no time.

What if I get depressed?

On a low-carb diet such as the Keto Zone, some people develop low serotonin levels, and that may bring on mild depression, feeling down, or food cravings. This typically occurs more often with women than men. An amino acid 5HTP (50 to 200 milligrams) or L-tryptophan (500 to 1000 milligrams) at bedtime will usually do wonders. Both are available at health food stores.

What if I am taking other medications?

One major benefit of the Keto Zone diet is the fact that your body will usually begin to heal in many ways. If you are taking medication for hypertension, diabetes, arthritis, or high cholesterol, you will need to follow up with your physician regularly to see if your dosage needs to be lowered or even discontinued.

What if I cannot sleep?

Make sure your last coffee or tea in the day is not after 2 or 3 p.m. That can interfere with sleep. Taking the amino acid 5HTP or L-tryptophan at night can help. One benefit of the Keto Zone diet is increased energy and, for many, a decreased need for sleep. When you sleep, it should be sound, but you may need less sleep as time progresses. Also try taking your magnesium supplement at bedtime since magnesium helps many with insomnia.

What is the worst that could happen to me?

Apart from the Keto Zone diet helping you uncover a medical issue (like gallstones) you already have, the diet usually should not cause you any harm. It is incredibly healthy, not to mention being the ideal way to lose weight. I do not recommend the Keto Zone diet for expectant mothers since it will prevent necessary weight gain during pregnancy.

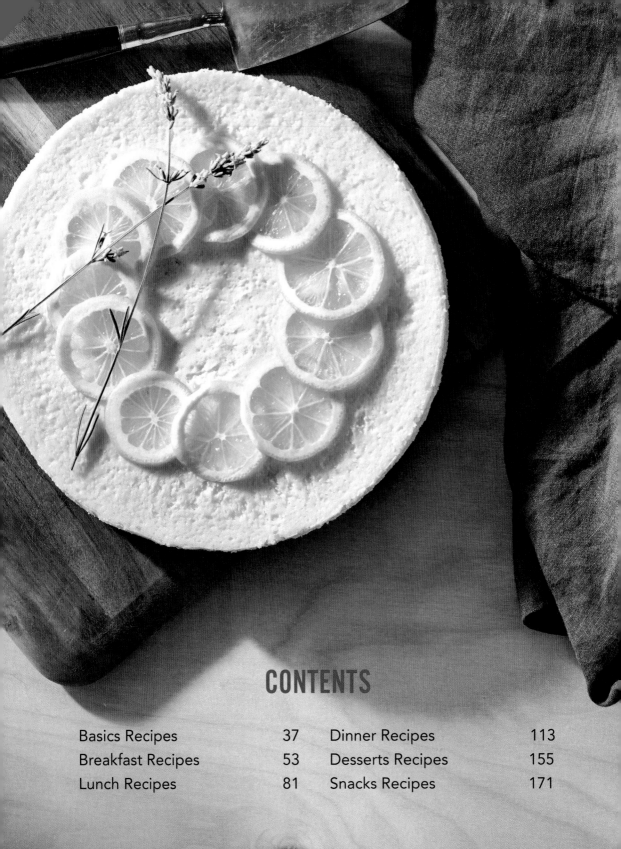

CONTENTS

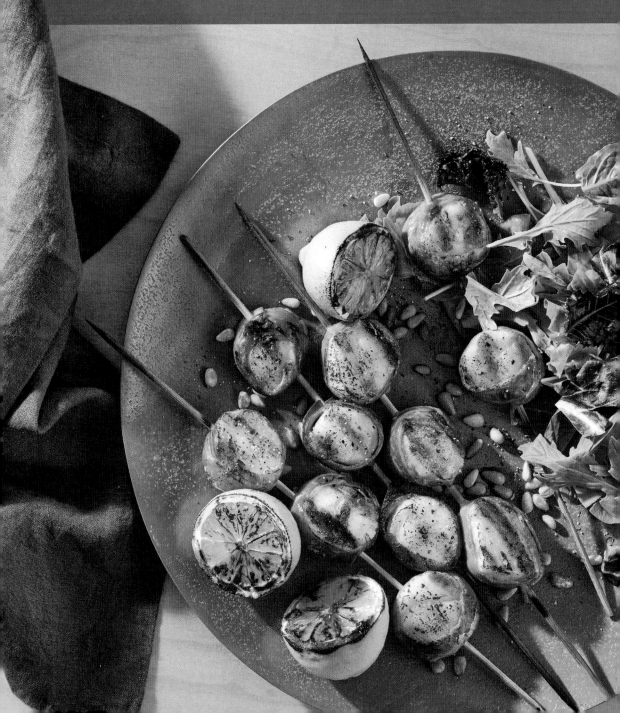

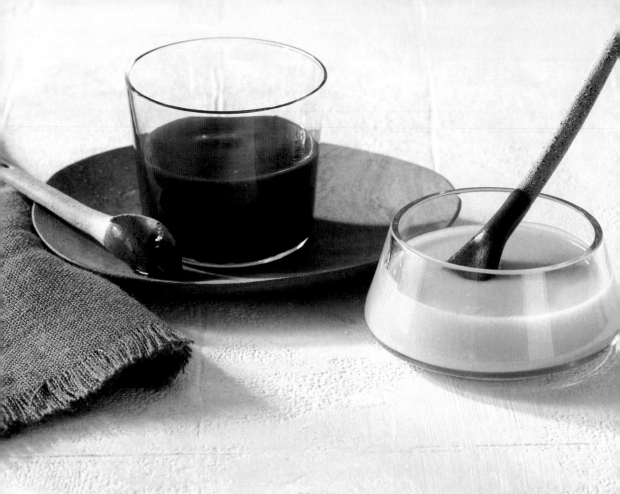

BASICS RECIPES

BASICS

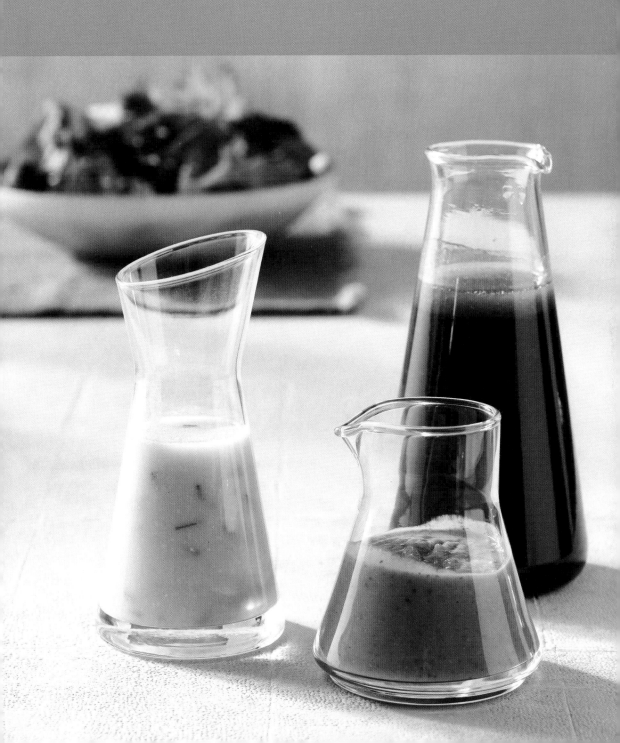

ALL DAY BONE BROTH

Yield: 4 quarts

With meat comes bones, and that's a good thing. This broth is a standard recipe that can be changed to fit any leftover bones you have. The easiest thing to do is store any bones and trimmings in a heavy-duty zip-top bag in the freezer until you have enough to use for this recipe. No need to thaw! Just take them straight to the slow cooker and let it simmer away all day.

6 grass-fed beef or pork bones*

2 celery stalks, cut in thirds

2 large garlic cloves, peeled and minced

1 onion, peeled and quartered

4 thyme sprigs

4 rosemary sprigs

4 peppercorns

1 bay leaf

2 tablespoons cider vinegar

2 teaspoons salt

4 quarts water

1 Place the bones* in the bottom of a large 6-quart slow cooker.

2 Add the celery, garlic, onion, thyme, rosemary, peppercorns, bay leaf, vinegar, and salt.

3 Add the water, cover, and cook on high for 1 hour.

4 After 1 hour, decrease the temperature to low and simmer 10 to 12 hours. Uncover and remove the insert from the slow cooker.

5 Allow to cool at least 1 hour before straining through a fine mesh colander. Discard the solids and refrigerate or freeze the broth.

*OPTION: To make chicken stock, substitute the pork bones for the carcass of 1 pastured, organic roasting chicken, along with skin and trimmed fat.

Serving size: 1 cup (beef or chicken)

calories	fat	protein	carbs	fiber
21	1.6g	0.19g	1.32g	0.32g

SLOW COOKER FISH STOCK

Yield: 4 quarts

Just like you would prepare bone broth, save the skin from low-mercury fish to make a delicate and very useful fish stock. Place the trimmings and leftovers in a heavy-duty zip-top bag in the freezer. When you have accumulated enough, pull out the slow cooker to get the process going. You can freeze the stock once it is finished.

6 cups fish trimmings

2 celery stalks, cut in thirds

1 onion, peeled and quartered

4 thyme sprigs

4 peppercorns

2 cloves

1 bay leaf

2 tablespoons cider vinegar

2 teaspoons salt

4 quarts water

1 Place the fish trimmings in the bottom of a large 6-quart slow cooker.

2 Add the celery, onion, thyme, peppercorns, cloves, bay leaf, vinegar, and salt.

3 Add the water, cover, and cook on low for 4 hours. Uncover and remove the insert from the slow cooker.

4 Allow to cool at least 1 hour before straining through a fine mesh colander. Discard the solids and refrigerate or freeze the stock.

Serving size: 1 cup

calories	fat	protein	carbs	fiber
52	5.14g	0.17g	1.26g	0.34g

COCONUT CREAM

Yield: 1⅓ cups

*Making your own coconut cream from coconut milk is incredibly easy.
Just make sure you purchase full-fat coconut milk
and your refrigerator does nearly all the work!*

1 (14.5-ounce) can
coconut milk
(It's best to find
a can made
without BPA.)

1 Place the unopened can of coconut milk in the
refrigerator at least 6 hours or overnight.

2 Remove from the refrigerator and immediately
turn the can upside down and open from the
bottom.

3 Pour out as much of the liquid as possible.
You will get around ¾ cup of liquid that can
be saved (refrigerated) for other cooking uses
or to use in smoothies.

4 The solid portion that is left is coconut cream.

COCONUT WHIPPED CREAM

Yield: ⅓ cup

1 Remove the thick coconut solids from the can
and transfer to the bowl of an electric mixer.
Beat until whipped like cream, about 2 minutes.

2 Use immediately, or store in an air tight
container for up to 2 days.

OPTIONAL: Add a few drops of liquid stevia for
added sweetness.

Serving size: ⅓ cup

calories	fat	protein	carbs	fiber
359	37.7g	3.9g	7.23g	2.39g

ALMOND LIME DIPPING SAUCE

Yield: ⅓ cup

This all-purpose sauce can be a salad dressing or grilled poultry dip.
Lime is an excellent addition for fish, poultry, or with mixed greens!

¼ cup liquid aminos

2 tablespoons
lime juice

2 tablespoons
almond oil

2 teaspoons
liquid stevia

¼ teaspoon
ground ginger

1 Place the liquid aminos, lime juice, oil, stevia, and ginger in a jar with a tight-fitting lid.

2 Shake well to emulsify.

3 Use immediately or refrigerate for up to 1 week.

calories	fat	protein	carbs	fiber
252	27g	7.7g	7.78g	0.34g

TARTAR SAUCE

Yield: 4 servings

This tartar sauce is enhanced with avocado mayonnaise.

½ teaspoon
onion salt

½ cup avocado
mayonnaise

1 gherkin pickle,
chopped

1 teaspoon
lemon juice

1 Stir together the salt, mayonnaise, pickle, and lemon juice.

2 Cover and refrigerate until ready to serve.

calories	fat	protein	carbs	fiber
206	22g	0.04g	1.41g	0.07g

MISTAKE-PROOF HOLLANDAISE SAUCE

Yield: ¾ cup

Hollandaise sauce is a classic usually served over poached eggs. Luckily, this favorite sauce is also Keto Zone-friendly and can be poured over meats or veggies to change up the flavor of another dish.

½ cup grass-fed butter (or ghee)

3 egg yolks

1 tablespoon + 1½ teaspoons lemon juice

¼ teaspoon salt

¼ teaspoon white pepper

1 Place the butter in a small saucepan over low heat to melt. Remove from heat to let cool slightly.

2 Meanwhile, place the egg yolks, lemon juice, salt, and pepper in a blender and process to combine.

3 With the blender speed on high, slowly add the slightly cooled melted butter through the lid opening.

4 Return to the saucepan, and keep warm until ready to use.

Serving size: ¼ cup

calories	fat	protein	carbs	fiber
341	35.4g	3.3g	5.33g	0.25g

CRÈME FRAÎCHE

Yield: 1 cup

*This thick cream has a really nice tangy flavor with a texture like silk.
You'll find multiple uses for it, especially in soups,
because it can be boiled without curdling.*

1 cup heavy whipping cream

2 tablespoons buttermilk or lemon juice

1 Stir together the cream and buttermilk in a glass container with a lid.

2 Cover and let stand at room temperature for at least 12 hours and up to 16 hours, until it's very thick.

3 Stir well, cover, and refrigerate.

4 Use within 1 week.

Serving size: ¼ cup

calories	fat	protein	carbs	fiber
207	21.7g	1.9g	2g	0g

TANGY BARBECUE SAUCE

Yield: 10 servings

This delicious sauce is perfect as is, but you can kick up the heat with the addition of more cayenne. Start with the smallest amount and adjust as you see fit.

2 medium tomatoes, peeled, seeded, and puréed

½ cup cider vinegar

¼ cup powdered erythritol

1½ tablespoons liquid aminos

1 tablespoon paprika

1 teaspoon garlic powder

½ teaspoon onion salt

¼ teaspoon black pepper

¼ to ½ teaspoon cayenne

1 In a medium saucepan over medium-high heat, stir together the tomato purée, vinegar, erythritol, liquid aminos, paprika, garlic powder, salt, pepper, and cayenne. Stir frequently until the mixture comes to a simmer.

2 Reduce heat to medium-low and simmer 15 minutes.

3 Remove from heat and cool to room temperature. If desired, add more cayenne.

4 Refrigerate if not using immediately.

calories	fat	protein	carbs	fiber
10.3	0.16g	0.66g	1.84g	0.6g

TZATZIKI

Yield: 3 servings

Traditionally served with Mediterranean dishes, this versatile sauce can be used as a dip with veggie chips or poured over any type of meat or alongside vegetables. Make the sauce at least the day before so the flavors have a chance to meld.

1 medium cucumber, grated

½ teaspoon salt

1 cup sour cream

1 large garlic clove, peeled and minced

1 tablespoon lemon juice

3 tablespoons olive oil

¼ teaspoon white pepper

1 tablespoon chopped fresh dill

1   Line a colander with paper towel or cheesecloth. Place the cucumber in the colander and sprinkle with salt. Let stand at room temperature 30 minutes.

2   Squeeze to remove any excess moisture and transfer to a medium mixing bowl.

3   Add the sour cream, garlic, lemon juice, oil, pepper, and dill. Stir well, cover, and refrigerate.

calories	fat	protein	carbs	fiber
290	28.5g	2.7g	8.15g	0.63g

GREEN GODDESS DRESSING

Yield: 4 servings

Green is the color of the day with dressing tossed with any salad greens.
It can be as thick or thin as you want by adjusting the amount of water used.

1 large avocado,
    peeled and pitted

1 large garlic clove,
    peeled

1 cup fresh
    basil leaves

¼ cup water or
    more for a thinner
    dressing

¼ cup avocado oil

2 tablespoons
    cider vinegar

1 teaspoon capers

¼ teaspoon salt

¼ teaspoon
    white pepper

1 Place the avocado, garlic, basil, water, oil,
   vinegar, capers, salt, and pepper in a blender
   and process until smooth.

2 Check the consistency and if a thinner dressing
   is desired, add 1 tablespoon of water at a time
   until the desired consistency is reached.

3 Serve tossed with mixed salad greens.
   Refrigerate any leftovers.

calories	fat	protein	carbs	fiber
206	21g	1.27g	4.9g	3.54g

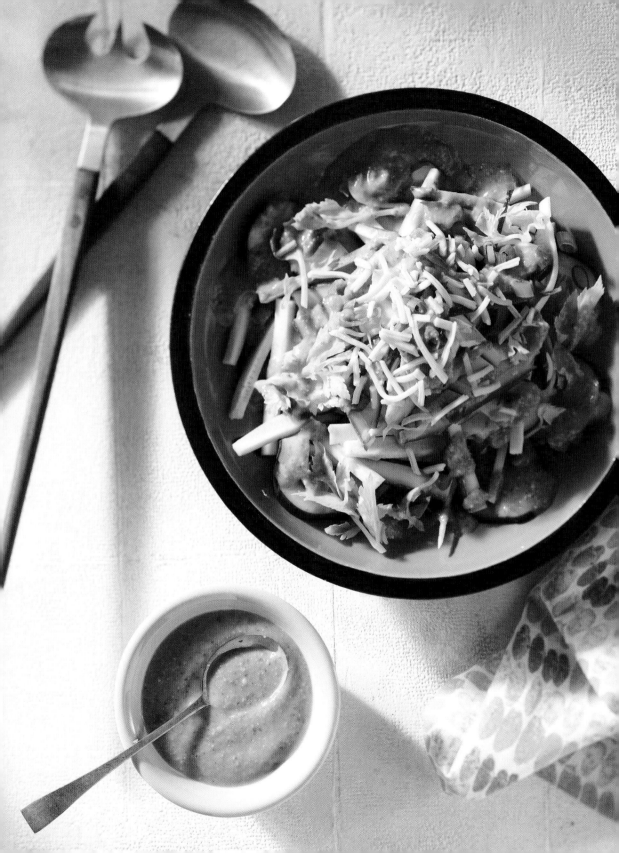

GINGER LIME DRESSING

Yield: 1⅓ cups

This dressing is made with liquid aminos, which looks and tastes like soy sauce, but has fewer carbs. At the store, you'll find it next to the soy sauce.

½ cup liquid aminos

⅓ cup lime juice

¼ cup cider vinegar

4 garlic cloves, peeled and minced

¾ cup avocado oil

2 tablespoons grated, peeled fresh ginger

1 Place the liquid aminos, lime juice, vinegar, garlic, oil, and ginger in a blender and process until smooth.

2 Transfer to a covered container, and refrigerate until ready to serve with mixed greens.

Serving size: ⅓ cup

calories	fat	protein	carbs	fiber
376	41g	4.1g	4.6g	0.2g

LEMON TAHINI DRESSING

Yield: ⅔ cup

Tahini lends just the right amount of nutty flavor and is especially nice with pork or on a salad.

¼ cup sour cream

¼ cup avocado mayonnaise

2 tablespoons tahini

1 tablespoon lemon juice

⅛ teaspoon white pepper

⅛ teaspoon cayenne

1 Place the sour cream, mayonnaise, tahini, lemon juice, pepper, and cayenne in a small bowl and whisk until smooth.

2 Drizzle over salad greens or store in a container in the refrigerator.

Serving size: ⅓ cup

calories	fat	protein	carbs	fiber
348	35.6g	3.37g	5.25g	0.8g

GARLIC HERB DRESSING

Yield: 1 cup

This dressing pairs perfectly with arugula, spinach, or a dark leafy green salad mix. Use any fresh herbs you like, such as parsley, tarragon, or chives.

½ cup avocado oil

¼ cup cider vinegar

3 garlic cloves, peeled

2 tablespoons water

1 tablespoon chopped fresh herbs

1½ teaspoons avocado mayonnaise

⅛ teaspoon salt

⅛ teaspoon white pepper

1 Place the oil, vinegar, garlic, water, herbs, mayonnaise, salt, and pepper in a food processor or blender and process until smooth.

2 Serve over salad greens, tossing thoroughly to coat the leaves. Refrigerate any leftovers.

Serving size: ¼ cup

calories	fat	protein	carbs	fiber
53	5.6g	0.1g	0.61g	0.33g

ITALIAN DRESSING

Yield: 2 servings

A healthier twist to this classic dressing.

¼ cup olive oil

2 tablespoons
cider vinegar

1 garlic clove, peeled
and minced

1 tablespoon grated
Romano or
Parmesan cheese

½ teaspoon
dried oregano

¼ teaspoon
onion salt

⅛ teaspoon
black pepper

1 In a jar with a tight-fitting lid, combine the oil, vinegar, garlic, Romano or Parmesan cheese, oregano, salt, and pepper.

2 Shake to emulsify and drizzle over salad greens or store in a container in the refrigerator.

calories	fat	protein	carbs	fiber
273	28.9g	2.4g	1.16g	0.17g

SALSA VERDE

Yields: 2 cups

Wanting to change up your lackluster weeknight dinner or need that extra something for a dinner party? Whip up this delicious sauce and you'll have people wiping the bowl clean. Drizzle over grilled or roasted meat and you've instantly upgraded your dish.

2 cups packed, roughly chopped flat leaf parsley

1 cup olive oil

¼ cup capers, drained

3 anchovy fillets (optional)

1½ tablespoons cider vinegar

1½ tablespoons lemon juice

2 medium garlic cloves, minced (about 2 teaspoons)

½ teaspoon freshly grated lemon zest (about 1 lemon, optional)

½ teaspoon salt

½ teaspoon freshly ground black pepper

1 Place parsley, olive oil, capers, anchovies (optional), vinegar, lemon juice, garlic, and lemon zest (optional) in the bowl of a food processor.

2 Pulse until all ingredients are well chopped, about 10 pulses, stopping to scrape down sides of bowl as necessary.

3 Season sauce with salt and pepper to taste. Transfer to a small bowl and let flavors meld together for 30 minutes to 1 hour. Stir once more and serve.

Serving size: ¼ cup

calories	fat	protein	carbs	fiber
251	27.3g	1.06g	1.92g	0.7g

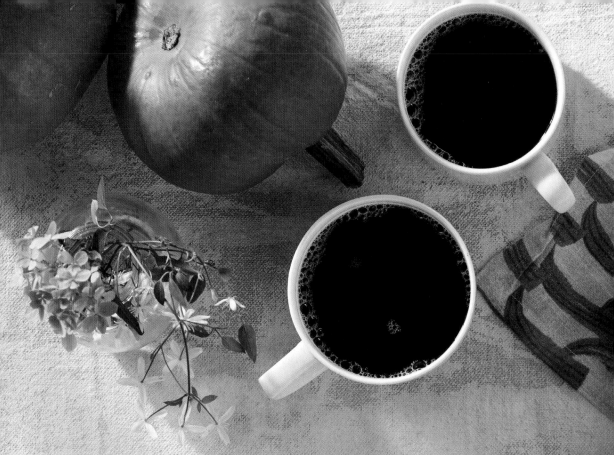

BREAKFAST RECIPES

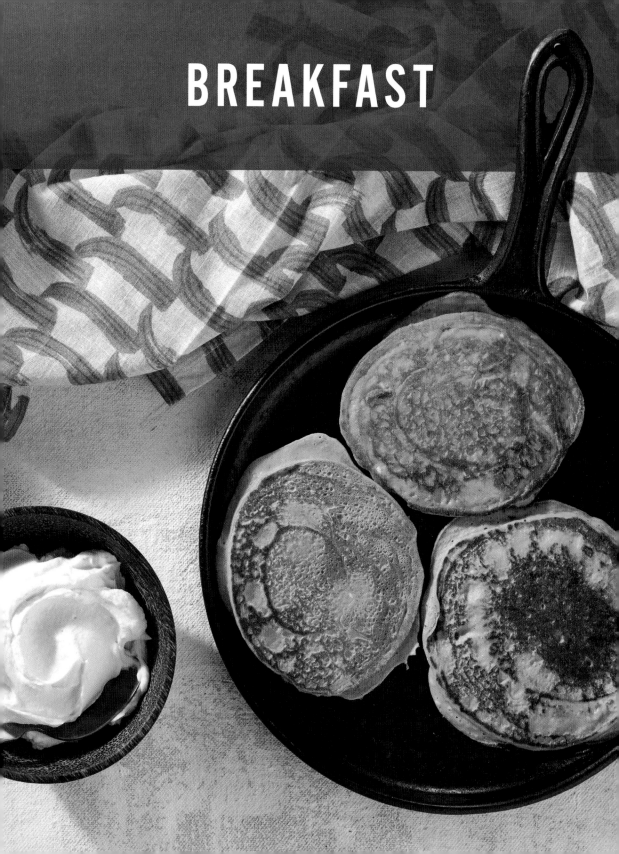

BREAKFAST

KETO ZONE COFFEE

Yield: 1 cup

Keto Zone Coffee is a meal in itself! The MCT oil powder gives you the fats you need to sustain you for three to five hours or longer. Jumpstart your day and stay in the Keto Zone with this quick drink.

8 to 12 ounces brewed hot coffee (ideally single-source)

1 tablespoon MCT oil powder

¼ teaspoon liquid stevia (optional)

1 tablespoon coconut oil or grass-fed butter (optional)

½ to 1 teaspoon unsweetened cocoa powder (optional)

1 Place the coffee, MCT oil powder, stevia (optional), oil or butter (optional), and cocoa powder (optional) into a blender.

2 Process until smooth. Process until the MCT powder and stevia are dissolved.

NOTE: Don't have time for the blender? You can briskly whisk the oil or butter, stevia, if using, and cocoa powder, if using, into your cup of hot coffee.

calories	fat	protein	carbs	fiber
197	21g	0.29g	0.62g	3.04g

SUNNY-SIDE UP EGGS (and variations!)

Yield: 1 serving

This classic is accomplished by cooking the eggs only on the bottom over low heat. See the notes below for other options.

2 to 3 tablespoons grass-fed butter (or ghee)

2 or 3 eggs

⅛ teaspoon salt

Pinch of black pepper

1 Place the butter in a skillet over medium-high heat.

2 When the butter has completely melted, tilt the skillet to coat the bottom of the pan.

3 Crack eggs and gently add to the skillet and immediately reduce the heat to low. Cook 3 minutes.

4 Sprinkle with the salt and pepper and serve immediately.

OVER-EASY EGGS: Flip the eggs over once with a large spatula after they have cooked for 3 minutes. Then season with the salt and pepper and serve.

OVER-WELL EGGS: After you have flipped the eggs, mash the eggs down with a spatula to break the yolks. Continue cooking another minute before seasoning with the salt and pepper.

calories	fat	protein	carbs	fiber
347	32.5g	12.8g	0.75g	0g

PERFECTLY SCRAMBLED EGGS

Yield: 2 servings

The key to moist scrambled eggs is to resist the temptation to stir them in the skillet constantly. You can change the taste by trying some of the flavor additions listed below.

1 to 2 tablespoon grass-fed butter (or ghee)

4 to 6 eggs

2 tablespoons unsweetened almond milk

¼ teaspoon salt

⅛ teaspoon black pepper

1   Place the butter in a skillet over medium heat.

2   When the butter has completely melted, tilt the skillet to coat the bottom of the pan.

3   Meanwhile, whisk together the eggs, milk, salt, and pepper.

4   Add the egg mixture and cook without stirring until the eggs begin to set on the bottom.

5   Draw the spatula across the bottom of the pan a few times to crumble.

6   Continue cooking until the eggs are thick and firm. Serve warm.

FLAVOR ADDITIONS: After step 6, stir to combine any of the following:

Add ¼ cup of shredded cheese

Add ¼ cup of diced onions, tomatoes, mushrooms, and garlic

Add ⅓ cup diced turkey sausage or ham

Add 1 tablespoon of chopped fresh herbs

calories	fat	protein	carbs	fiber
222	18.3g	12.8g	0.91g	0.04g

POACHED EGGS

Yield: 2 servings

Poaching is a cooking method that allows eggs to cook in barely simmering water. If you have poaching cups, the process is easy! Serve with Mistake-Proof Hollandaise Sauce (page 42).

WITHOUT POACHING CUPS:

4 to 6 eggs

1 Lightly grease a wide saucepan with olive oil cooking spray. Add enough water so the depth is 2 inches.

2 Place over high heat and bring the water nearly to a boil. Reduce heat to low to maintain a low simmer.

3 Break the eggs, one at a time, into a measuring cup and holding the cup as close to the water's surface as possible, slip the egg into the water.

4 Repeat with the remaining eggs.

5 Simmer 5 minutes and remove the cooked eggs with a slotted spoon. Serve immediately.

WITH POACHING CUPS:

4 to 6 eggs

1 Lightly grease each cup with olive oil cooking spray. Place the poacher tray in a pan of simmering water. The water should be below the bottom of the tray.

2 Break an egg into each cup.

3 Cover and cook 5 minutes.

4 Using the cup handles, slip the eggs onto a plate and serve immediately.

calories	fat	protein	carbs	fiber
143	9.5g	12.5g	0.71g	0g

SHIRRED EGGS

Yield: 4 servings

If you really want a nice presentation, your oven is the place to go for preparing eggs. Shirred eggs are baked in small dishes so each person has their own container. Traditionally, the whites are firm and the yolks are still a little soft, but you can adjust the cooking time to suit your own taste.

4 large, extra large, or jumbo eggs

¼ teaspoon salt

⅛ teaspoon black pepper

4 tablespoons heavy whipping cream

1 Preheat the oven to 325 degrees.

2 Lightly grease four 6-ounce custard cups with olive oil cooking spray. Place cups on a rimmed baking sheet.

3 Break one egg into each cup and sprinkle evenly with salt and pepper.

4 Spoon 1 tablespoon cream on top of each egg.

5 Carefully transfer baking sheet to the oven and bake uncovered for 15 minutes. Serve immediately.

calories	fat	protein	carbs	fiber
123	10.2g	6.71g	0.82g	0.02g

HARD-BOILED EGGS

Yield: 4 servings

Hard-boiled eggs is a classic must have recipe.

4 to 6 large, extra large or jumbo eggs

1 Place the eggs in a medium saucepan and add enough cold water to cover by 1 inch.

2 Place over medium-high heat. As soon as the water comes to a boil, remove from the heat and cover. Let stand 15 minutes.

3 Drain and transfer the eggs to a bowl of ice water. Let stand until cool. Peel the eggs.

calories	fat	protein	carbs	fiber
77	5.3g	6.3g	0.56g	0g

BASIC OMELET

Yield: 1 serving

The same techniques used to make scrambled eggs are used for making omelets. The difference is that an omelet is folded over the fillings rather than having the additions mixed throughout the eggs. Once you have mastered the art of an omelet, you have a whole world of possibilities for fillings.

1 tablespoon
   grass-fed butter
   (or ghee)

2 to 3 eggs

1 tablespoon water
   or avocado oil

⅛ teaspoon salt

Pinch of black pepper

1 In a mixing bowl whisk together the eggs, water, salt, and pepper.

2 Place the butter in a heavy skillet over medium heat. When the butter has completely melted, tilt the skillet to coat the bottom of the pan.

3 Pour the egg mixture into the pan.

4 As the eggs cook, gently lift up the edges with a spatula and tilt the pan so the uncooked portion slides underneath. It will all cook in 2 minutes or less.

5 Sprinkle the desired filling ingredients over half of the eggs. Fold the omelet in half to cover the fillings. Cook another 1 to 2 minutes to heat filling. Serve immediately.

FILLING OPTIONS: (pick 1 meat and up to 2 other options)

2 slices cooked and crumbled turkey bacon

2 tablespoons diced ham or turkey sausage

2 tablespoons grated cheese

1 tablespoon diced onion, 1 tablespoon diced tomatoes, 1 tablespoon diced mushrooms, and ½ minced garlic clove

1 tablespoon chopped fresh herbs

2 to 3 ounce spinach

¼ to ½ sliced avocado added on finished omelet

calories	fat	protein	carbs	fiber
245	21g	12.7g	0.79g	0.03g

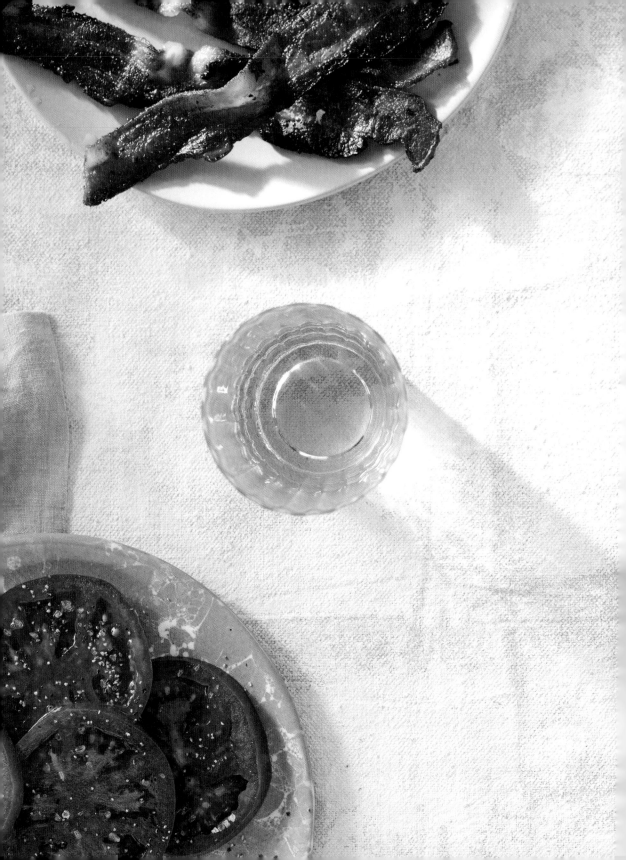

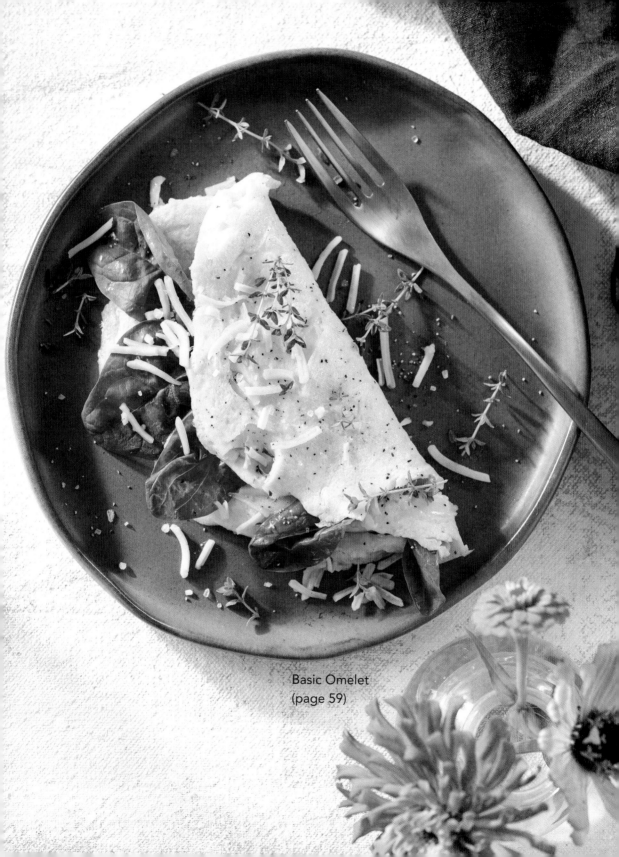

Basic Omelet
(page 59)

PUFFED OMELET

Yield: 2 servings

The oven is essential for this impressive dish. The eggs are separated so the egg whites can be beaten. This gives the omelet the air it needs to puff up beautifully. Top with any cheese or herbs you like, or enjoy it plain.

4 to 6 eggs, separated

2 tablespoons heavy whipping cream

¼ teaspoon salt

⅛ teaspoon black pepper

1 tablespoon grass-fed butter (or ghee)

2 tablespoons grated cheese or cream cheese

1 tablespoon fresh parsley, chopped

1 Preheat the oven to 325 degrees.

2 Place the egg whites in the bowl of an electric mixer and beat at medium speed until frothy.

3 Add the cream, salt, and pepper and continue beating at medium-high speed until stiff peaks form.

4 In a separate bowl, beat the yolks with a fork and gently fold into the egg whites.

5 Place the butter in a large, ovenproof skillet over medium heat. When the butter has completely melted, tilt the skillet to evenly coat the bottom.

6 With a spatula, spread the egg mixture in the pan, making sure the sides are higher than the middle.

7 Cover and reduce the heat to low. Cook 5 to 7 minutes or until puffed.

8 Uncover and transfer the skillet to the oven. Bake 10 minutes or until a knife inserted in the center comes out clean.

9 With a spatula, loosen one side of the omelet and fold over the other half. Gently slide onto a serving plate and top immediately with the cheese and parsley. Serve warm.

calories	fat	protein	carbs	fiber
297	25.7g	14g	2.24g	0.14g

CREAM CHEESE SCRAMBLED EGGS

Yield: 3 servings

It is amazing how the addition of just a bit of cream cheese changes the texture and flavor of ordinary scrambled eggs.

3 tablespoons grass-fed butter (or ghee)

6 to 9 eggs

½ cup unsweetened almond milk

3 ounces cream cheese, cubed

2 tablespoons fresh chives or parsley, chopped

¼ teaspoon salt

⅛ teaspoon black pepper

1 Place the eggs, milk, cream cheese, herbs, salt, and pepper in a blender and process until smooth.

2 Meanwhile, place the butter in a large skillet over medium heat. When the butter has completely melted, tilt the skillet to evenly coat the bottom.

3 Pour the egg mixture into the skillet and cook without stirring for 1 to 2 minutes or until the mixture begins to set on the bottom.

4 Drag the spatula across the bottom of the skillet two or three times to crumble and continue cooking without stirring until the eggs are thick. Serve warm.

calories	fat	protein	carbs	fiber
351	31.3g	14.8g	2.7g	0.07g

BAKED EGGS WITH CITRUS CREAM

Yield: 2 to 4 servings

This trick of pairing cream with citrus juice has been used for years by chefs to add interest without using sugar. Here it works quite nicely with eggs for a memorable breakfast.

2 green onions, chopped

1 tablespoon chopped fresh parsley

2 to 4 eggs

1 tablespoon grass-fed butter, melted

¼ cup heavy whipping cream

Juice of ½ small orange

1 tablespoon lemon juice

¼ teaspoon salt

⅛ teaspoon black pepper

1 Preheat the oven to 325 degrees.

2 Lightly grease 2 to 4 small ramekins with the melted butter and sprinkle the onions and parsley over the bottoms.

3 Carefully break an egg into each ramekin, being careful not to break the yolks.

4 In a glass measuring cup, whisk together the cream, orange juice, and lemon juice.

5 Gently pour half the mixture over each egg and sprinkle with the salt and pepper.

6 Bake 15 to 17 minutes or until the eggs are set.

7 Allow to cool 5 minutes before serving warm.

	calories	fat	protein	carbs	fiber
	138	10.3g	7.04g	4.37g	0.35g

SPRING GREEN QUICHE

Yield: 6 servings

*Make this substantial breakfast on Sunday morning, then enjoy
the reheated leftovers to start your weekday. If desired, you can use
only spinach or kale rather than a combination.*

3 tablespoons
avocado oil

2 cups kale, chopped

1 cup spinach,
chopped

5 eggs

2 tablespoons
unsweetened
almond milk

2 garlic cloves, peeled
and minced

½ teaspoon
black pepper

½ teaspoon salt

⅛ teaspoon cayenne

1 cup grated
Gruyère cheese

1 Preheat the oven to 350 degrees.

2 Lightly grease a 9-inch pie pan with olive oil
cooking spray and set aside.

3 Place the oil in a large skillet over
medium-high heat.

4 Add the kale and cook 3 minutes.

5 Add the spinach and continue cooking
3 minutes, stirring to wilt the greens.

6 Set aside to cool slightly.

7 In a large mixing bowl, whisk the eggs
until frothy.

8 Add the milk, garlic, pepper, salt, and cayenne,
whisking thoroughly to combine.

9 Stir in the greens and Gruyère cheese.

10 Transfer to the prepared pie pan and bake
40 minutes or until knife inserted in middle
comes out clean.

11 Allow to rest 5 minutes before slicing and
serving.

calories	fat	protein	carbs	fiber
203	16.9g	11.1g	1.5g	0.38g

ITALIAN FRITTATA

Yield: 6 servings

This breakfast is made for weekends or holidays. Unlike omelets that are cooked quickly over high heat, frittatas are cooked over low heat, are finished in the oven, and are not folded. It is an Italian specialty, and signature ingredients are added to give it flavor.

1 pound baby spinach, chopped

8 eggs

3 tablespoons grated Parmesan cheese

2 tablespoons heavy whipping cream

2 tablespoons chopped sun-dried tomatoes

½ teaspoon onion salt

¼ teaspoon black pepper

4 tablespoons avocado oil

2 garlic cloves, peeled and minced

1 shallot, peeled and minced

¼ cup crumbled feta cheese

1　Preheat the oven to 400 degrees.

2　In a large mixing bowl, whisk together the eggs, Parmesan cheese, cream, tomatoes, salt, and pepper.

3　Place the oil in a large, ovenproof skillet over medium-high heat.

4　Add the garlic and shallot and cook, stirring constantly, for 2 minutes.

5　Reduce the heat to medium-low and add the spinach, spreading evenly across the bottom of the skillet.

6　Pour the egg mixture over the top and sprinkle with the feta cheese.

7　Cook undisturbed for 3 minutes or until the egg mixture is set on the bottom, but still runny on the top.

8　Transfer to the oven and bake for 15 to 20 minutes or until the frittata is puffed and golden brown.

9　Let stand 5 minutes before slicing and serving.

	calories	fat	protein	carbs	fiber
	256	20.1g	12.8g	7.14g	2.27g

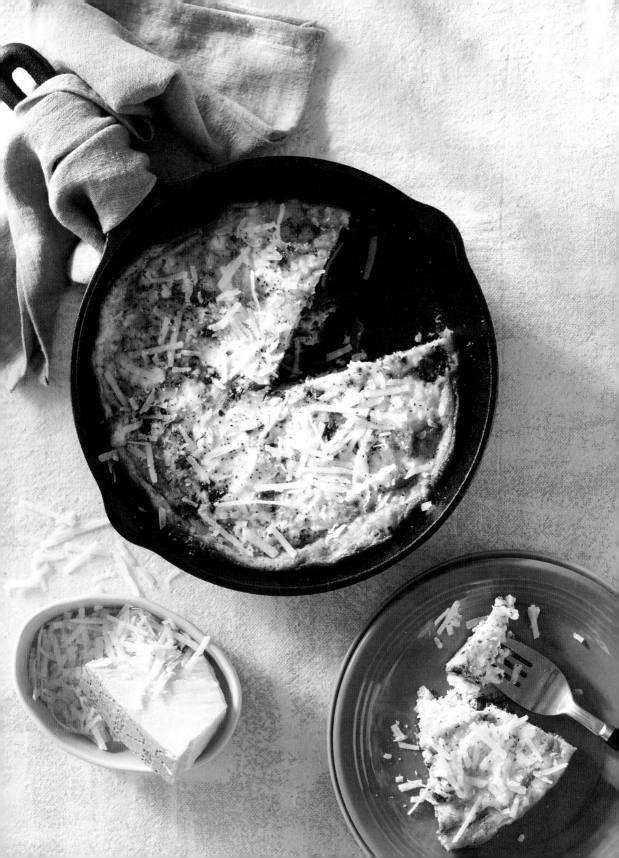

BRUSSELS SPROUTS EGG PIE

Yield: 3 to 4 servings

This versatile breakfast can be made using any number of cruciferous vegetables, such as radishes, bok choy, cauliflower, or broccoli. Try it first with the brussels sprouts, then get creative!

3 tablespoons avocado oil

1 cup thinly sliced brussels sprouts

6 eggs

2 garlic cloves, peeled and minced

⅓ cup unsweetened almond milk

½ cup Muenster cheese

2 tablespoons chopped fresh parsley

1 tablespoon chopped fresh chives

1 teaspoon chopped fresh rosemary

½ teaspoon white pepper

½ teaspoon salt

1 Preheat the oven to 350 degrees.

2 Lightly grease a 9-inch pie pan with olive oil cooking spray and set aside.

3 Place the oil in a large skillet over medium-high heat.

4 When the pan is hot, add the brussels sprouts and cook for 4 minutes or until soft.

5 Set aside to cool slightly.

6 In a large mixing bowl, whisk the eggs until frothy.

7 Add the garlic, milk, Muenster cheese, parsley, chives, rosemary, pepper, and salt.

8 Stir in the brussels sprouts and transfer to the prepared pie pan.

9 Bake 35 minutes or knife inserted in center comes out clean.

10 Allow to rest 5 minutes before slicing and serving.

calories	fat	protein	carbs	fiber
360	29.6g	18.5g	5.19g	1.51g

TURKEY IMPERIAL

Yield: 3 servings

*Assemble your ingredients the night before, then stir together
and allow to bake while you get ready for work.
You'll have a weekend-worthy breakfast that will help you face the day!*

3 eggs

3 tablespoons
avocado mayonnaise

2 tablespoons
sour cream

2 tablespoons
grass-fed butter,
melted

1 teaspoon lemon juice

¼ teaspoon
garlic salt

¼ teaspoon cayenne

¼ teaspoon
black pepper

½ pound ground
turkey, cooked*

1 teaspoon paprika

2 tablespoons
slivered almonds*

1 Preheat the oven to 350 degrees.

2 Lightly grease 3 ramekins with olive oil cooking
spray and place on a baking sheet. Set aside.

3 In a mixing bowl, whisk together the eggs,
mayonnaise, sour cream, butter, lemon juice,
salt, cayenne, and pepper. Stir in the turkey.

4 Spoon evenly into the prepared ramekins and
sprinkle with the paprika. Bake 20 minutes or
until light brown on top.

5 Remove from the oven and immediately top
with the slivered almonds.

6 Allow to rest 5 minutes before serving warm.

*NOTE: Substitute cooked ground chicken or diced
ham for the turkey, if desired. Also, finely grated
sharp Cheddar cheese can be substituted for the
almonds.

calories	fat	protein	carbs	fiber
450	39g	21.4g	3.64g	1.42g

SMOKED SALMON MINI CRUSTLESS QUICHES

Yield: 6 mini quiches

The secret ingredient for these scrumptious mini quiches is crème fraîche (page 43). If necessary, you can substitute heavy whipping cream. These freeze beautifully.

3 ½ ounces chopped smoked salmon

2 green onions, chopped

2 teaspoons chopped fresh dill

5 eggs

5 teaspoons crème fraîche (page 43)

¼ teaspoon salt

¼ teaspoon black pepper

1 Preheat the oven to 325 degrees. Lightly grease 6 muffin cups with olive oil cooking spray or line with paper liners. Evenly divide the salmon, onions, and dill in each of the 6 cups. Set aside.

2 In a mixing bowl, whisk together the eggs, crème fraîche, salt, and pepper.

3 Pour into the muffin cups, filling them three-quarters full.

4 Bake 13 to 15 minutes or knife inserted in center comes out clean.

5 Cool completely on a wire rack. Serve at room temperature.

Serving size: 1 quiche

calories	fat	protein	carbs	fiber
129	7.1g	15.4g	0.71g	0.1g

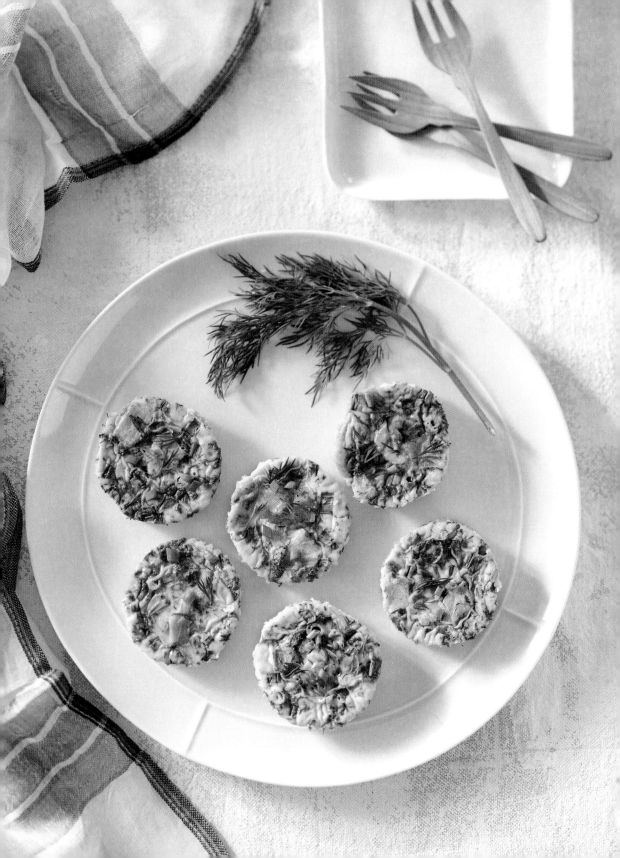

ALMOND FLAXSEED WAFFLES

Yield: 4 waffles

This may be your new go-to Saturday morning breakfast!
Ground flaxseeds may be labeled "flaxseed meal" at the supermarket.

¾ cup unsweetened almond milk

1 tablespoon almond oil

1½ teaspoons liquid stevia

1 teaspoon pure almond extract

¾ teaspoon cider vinegar

½ cup almond or coconut flour

¾ teaspoon baking powder

¼ teaspoon baking soda

Pinch of salt

1½ tablespoons ground flaxseeds

¼ cup slivered almonds

1 Place the milk, almond oil, stevia, almond extract, and vinegar in a blender and combine. Let stand 10 minutes.

2 Meanwhile, in a medium mixing bowl, stir together the flour, baking powder, baking soda, and salt. Set aside.

3 Add the flaxseeds to the milk mixture and blend for 1 minute.

4 Spray a waffle iron with olive oil cooking spray and preheat.

5 Add the milk mixture to the flour mixture and stir and stir just until combined. Fold in the almonds.

6 Use about ⅓ cup of batter to make each waffle. Cook according to the manufacturer's directions until golden brown. Serve warm.

FRUIT SYRUP (OPTIONAL)

1 cup raspberries or strawberries

4 tablespoons grass-fed butter

1 Make a syrup by simmering the berries with the butter until the berries begin to release their juices.

Serving size: 1 waffle (no topping)

calories	fat	protein	carbs	fiber
216	19.2g	6.67g	8.15g	3.84g

SAVORY BREAKFAST MUFFINS

Yield: 5 muffins

Cheese muffins are terrific in the morning. If you have some leftover chopped spinach or kale, fold a half-cup into the batter. Cooked, chopped mushrooms are a good addition as well.

½ cup almond flour

½ teaspoon baking powder

⅛ teaspoon garlic or onion salt

⅛ teaspoon black pepper

⅛ teaspoon cayenne

⅛ teaspoon paprika

2 eggs

⅓ cup small-curd whole-fat cottage cheese

1 tablespoon grated Parmesan cheese

1 tablespoon chopped fresh parsley

¼ cup crumbled feta cheese

1 chopped green onion

1 Preheat the oven to 400 degrees.

2 Lightly grease 5 muffin cups with olive oil cooking spray, or fill with paper liners and set aside.

3 In a large mixing bowl, stir together the flour, baking powder, salt, pepper, cayenne, and paprika.

4 Make a well in the center of the flour mixture and stir in the eggs, cottage cheese, Parmesan cheese, and parsley.

5 Fold in the feta cheese and green onions, stirring just until blended.

6 Divide the batter evenly among the muffin cups.

7 Bake 22 to 24 minutes or until the tops are golden brown.

8 Cool in the pan for 3 minutes before serving warm or transfer to a wire rack to cool completely.

Serving size: 1 muffin

calories	fat	protein	carbs	fiber
133	10.1g	8g	3.9g	1.32g

PUMPKIN PANCAKES

Yield: 9 pancakes

This recipe works great for company or family gatherings.
Serve it with Coconut Cream or Coconut Whipped Cream (page 40).

1 cup canned unsweetened pumpkin purée (not pumpkin pie filling)

8 ounces (1 cup) cream cheese, softened

1 cup coconut flour

3 eggs

¼ cup grass-fed butter, melted

1 to 2 drops liquid stevia

½ teaspoon pumpkin pie spice

2 tablespoons coconut oil, divided

1 In a large mixing bowl, combine the pumpkin purée, cream cheese, flour, eggs, butter, stevia, and pumpkin pie spice. Blend well and set aside for 20 minutes.

2 Preheat the oven to 200 degrees.

3 Place 1 tablespoon coconut oil in a large skillet over medium heat.

4 When the skillet is hot, spoon the batter in the skillet and cook until small bubbles form around the edges and on top of each pancake. Flip and cook until golden brown.

5 Place pancakes on a baking sheet, cover with foil, and place in the oven to keep warm.

6 Add remaining coconut oil to the skillet when half the batter has been used. Repeat cooking pancakes until all the batter has been used.

7 Serve warm with coconut cream, coconut whipped cream (page 40), or fruit syrup (page 72).

Serving size: 1 pancake (no topping)

calories	fat	protein	carbs	fiber
271	20.4g	5.8g	16.7g	6.95g

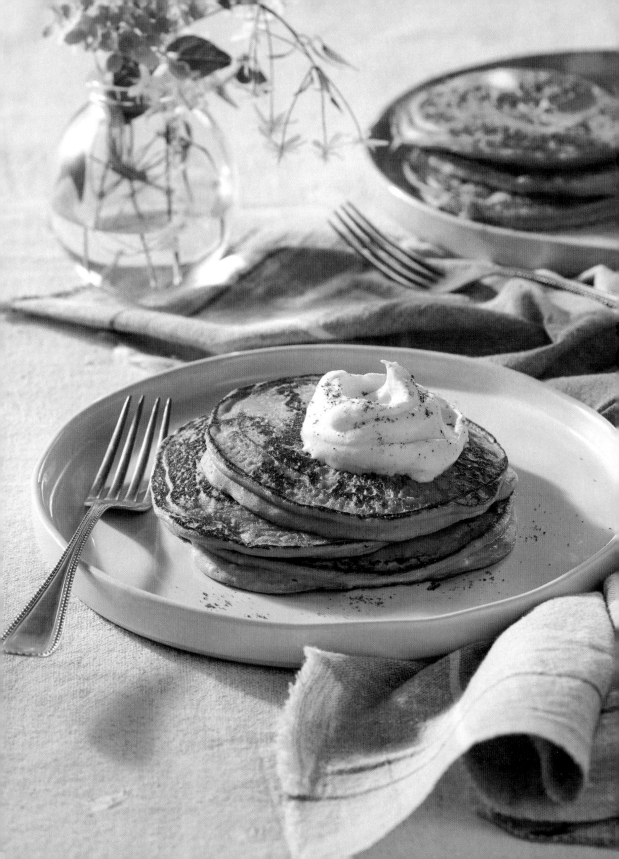

ALMOND COCONUT CEREAL

Yield: 4 to 5 servings

Make this cereal mixture over the weekend and you will have breakfast made for the work week. Store in an airtight container in the refrigerator.

3 cups unsweetened shredded or flaked coconut

1 cup sliced or slivered almonds

1 tablespoon pure almond extract

1 tablespoon ground cinnamon

½ teaspoon powdered stevia

1 Preheat the oven to 300 degrees, and lightly coat a rimmed baking sheet with olive oil cooking spray.

2 Spread the coconut and almonds on the baking sheet and sprinkle with the almond extract. Toss gently to coat, and spread evenly on the baking sheet.

3 Bake 5 minutes or until lightly browned.

4 Place the baking sheet on a wire rack and sprinkle evenly with the cinnamon and stevia.

5 Stir well and cool to room temperature. Serve with unsweetened almond or coconut milk.

calories	fat	protein	carbs	fiber
384	33.3g	12.1g	14.9g	8.29g

FROZEN BERRY SMOOTHIE

Yield: 1 serving

*This simple shake is packed with nutrients and utilizes the ease
of frozen strawberries. See the variations below.*

6 to 8 ounces
  unsweetened
  almond or
  coconut milk

1 tablespoon
  MCT oil powder

¼ cup frozen
  strawberries

1 tablespoon
  almond butter

1 tablespoon coconut
  or avocado oil

¼ teaspoon
  liquid stevia

1 Place the milk, protein powder, strawberries,
   almond butter, coconut or avocado oil, and
   stevia in a blender.

2 Process until smooth. Enjoy immediately.

RASPBERRY SMOOTHIE: Substitute ¼ cup frozen
raspberries for the strawberries.

BLUEBERRY SMOOTHIE: Use coconut milk and
substitute macadamia butter for the almond
butter, and ¼ cup frozen blueberries instead of
the strawberries.

BLACKBERRY SMOOTHIE: Substitute pecan or peanut
butter for the almond butter and ¼ cup frozen
blackberries for the strawberries.

calories	fat	protein	carbs	fiber
367	32.2g	5.07g	15.5g	7.98g

CHOCOLATE PEANUT SMOOTHIE

Yield: 1 serving

*Enjoy this delicious blend of chocolate and peanut butter
for breakfast or dessert!*

6 to 8 ounces
unsweetened
almond or
coconut milk

1 scoop
MCT oil powder

1 tablespoon organic,
unsweetened
peanut butter

1 tablespoon coconut
or avocado oil

1 teaspoon
unsweetened cocoa

¼ teaspoon
liquid stevia

1 Place the milk, protein powder, peanut butter,
coconut or avocado oil, cocoa, and stevia in
a blender.

2 Process until smooth.

3 Add 3 ice cubes and process until the ice is
crushed. Enjoy immediately.

calories	fat	protein	carbs	fiber
326	31.5g	5.27g	6.56g	4.5g

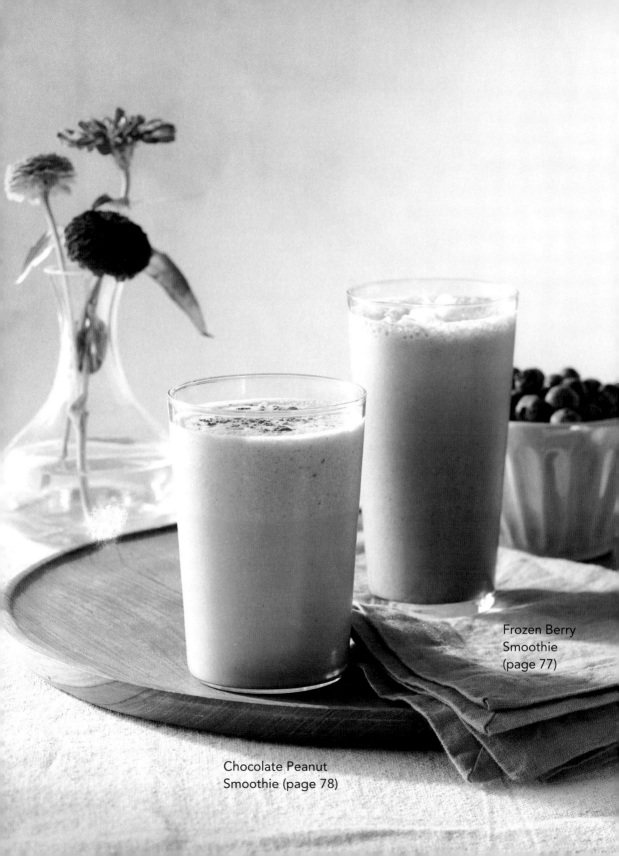

Frozen Berry
Smoothie
(page 77)

Chocolate Peanut
Smoothie (page 78)

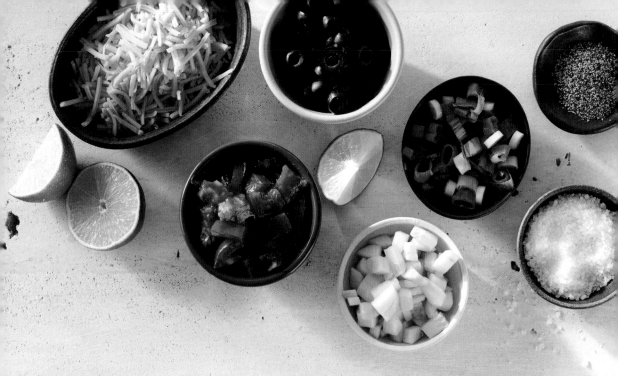

LUNCH RECIPES

LUNCH

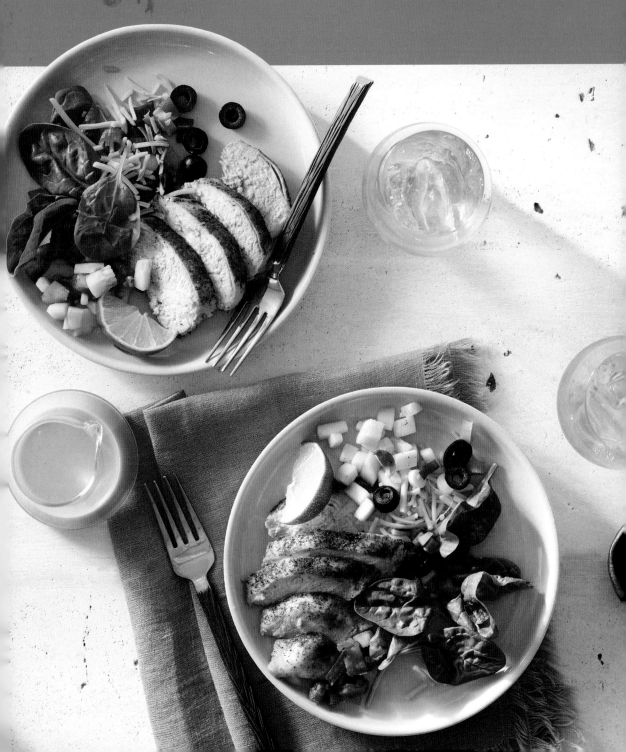

ROASTED CAULIFLOWER & CRAB SOUP

Yield: 6 to 8 servings

This soup is rich, creamy, and totally satisfying.
This soup freezes well, but freeze the crab and soup separately.
Thaw both and continue step 9 when thawed.

1 large head
cauliflower, trimmed
and cut into florets

10 tablespoons
avocado oil, divided

½ teaspoon
garlic salt, divided

¼ teaspoon
black pepper

2 shallots, peeled and
chopped

2 teaspoons cumin

2 cups chicken stock
(page 38)

4 cups water

1 pound
lump crab meat

1 tablespoon
lemon juice

Chopped fresh chives
for garnish

1   Preheat the oven to 350 degrees.

2   Place the cauliflower florets on a lightly greased
baking sheet.

3   Drizzle with 2 tablespoons oil, and sprinkle on
¼ teaspoon salt and pepper. Roast 25 minutes,
turning the florets halfway through the cooking
process.

4   Meanwhile, place 2 tablespoons oil in a Dutch
oven medium-high heat.

5   Add the shallots and cook 6 minutes, stirring
frequently.

6   Sprinkle with the cumin and remaining
¼ teaspoon salt. Cook 1 minute longer,
stirring constantly.

7   Add the chicken stock and water. When the
mixture comes to a boil, add the cauliflower,
cover, and reduce the heat to low. Simmer,
stirring occasionally, for 20 minutes.

8   Add remaining oil, and with an immersion
blender, purée the soup until smooth.

9   Stir in the crab meat and lemon juice and heat
an additional minute. Serve warm with a garnish
of chopped fresh chives.

calories	fat	protein	carbs	fiber
309	22.3g	17.6g	11.2g	3.17g

SHRIMP & CUCUMBER SOUP

Yield: 6 servings

Cold soup on a hot day is a great way to cool down.
This recipe can be made quickly the day before if necessary.

2 large cucumbers, peeled, seeded, and coarsely chopped

1 green onion, chopped

1 tablespoon lemon juice

1 (18-ounce) container sour cream

1 cup half-and-half

1 tablespoon fresh dill, minced

1 teaspoon salt

½ teaspoon white pepper

⅛ teaspoon hot sauce

2 cups cooked salad shrimp

Fresh dill sprigs for garnish

1 Process the cucumbers, onion, and lemon juice in a food processor until the mixture is smooth. Transfer to a large mixing bowl.

2 Add the sour cream, half-and-half, minced dill, salt, pepper, and hot sauce, stirring well to blend.

3 Fold in the shrimp, cover, and refrigerate at least 2 hours.

4 Serve in chilled soup bowls and garnish with fresh dill sprigs.

calories	fat	protein	carbs	fiber
310	20g	23.7g	8.61g	0.76g

AVOCADO SOUP

Yield: 6 servings

This is the recipe to use if you have avocados that are not quite ripe. The heat allows them to become softer and more flavorful.

4 cups bone broth (page 38), divided

1 small onion, peeled and chopped

4 green onions, sliced

2 garlic cloves, peeled and minced

½ teaspoon garlic salt

¼ teaspoon black pepper

Pinch of ground nutmeg (optional)

4 tablespoons avocado oil

2 zucchini, thinly sliced

2 avocados, pitted, peeled, and chopped

1 Place 1 cup of the bone broth in a large pot over medium-high heat.

2 When steaming, add the onion, green onions, garlic, salt, pepper, and nutmeg, if desired. Bring to a boil, cover, and reduce heat to low. Cook 15 minutes.

3 Add the remaining 3 cups broth, oil, and zucchini; increase heat to medium-high. Bring to a boil, stirring occasionally. Cover and reduce heat to low. Cook 20 minutes.

4 Stir in the avocados.

5 With an immersion blender, purée until smooth. Serve warm.

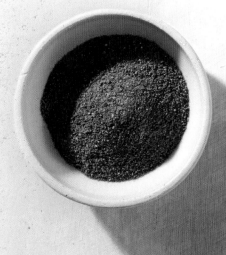

calories	fat	protein	carbs	fiber
267	21.3g	6.4g	15.3g	5.53g

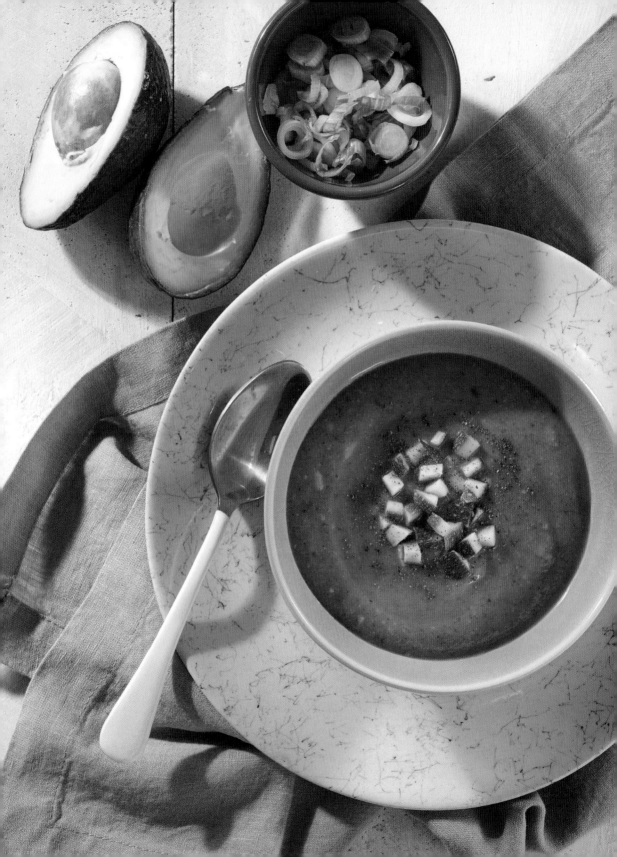

CHICKEN ZOODLE SOUP

Yields: 8 servings

This is an excellent Keto friendly soup for when you're craving a hearty soup. Spiralized zucchini noodles are the perfect substitute for flour noodles.

10 tablespoons avocado oil, divided

3 tablespoons grass-fed butter, softened

5 cups chicken stock (see page 38)

4 organic pastured boneless, chicken breasts (about 5 cups)

4 to 5 large zucchini

3 garlic cloves, minced

1 small onion, chopped

8 to 10 asparagus stalks, chopped

6 celery stalks, chopped

½ teaspoon ground turmeric

4 teaspoons dried basil, finely chopped

4 teaspoons dried parsley, finely chopped

2 bay leaves

2 teaspoons sea salt, divided

2 teaspoons black pepper, divided

1 Preheat the oven to 375 degrees.

2 Rub softened butter all over chicken breasts and season with 1 teaspoon of salt and pepper. Place chicken breasts in a roasting pan, skin side up.

3 Roast chicken for 15 minutes, then flip chicken and bake another 10 to12 minutes, or until chicken is no longer pink.

4 Remove from oven and let cool slightly before removing skin and dicing, yielding about 5 cups.

5 In a Dutch oven or large soup pot, heat 5 tablespoons of oil over medium-high heat.

6 Add onion, celery, and asparagus, and cook, stirring often, until vegetables have softened, about 5 minutes. Add garlic and cook for additional minute.

7 Add chicken stock, turmeric, basil, parsley, salt, pepper, bay leaves, 5 tablespoons of oil, and chopped chicken.

8 Bring to a boil and reduce to low heat. Simmer, stirring occasionally for 30 minutes.

9 While soup simmers, spiralize the zucchini.

10 Remove pot from heat and stir in zucchini noodles. Let sit for about 10 minutes until zoodles soften.

11 Remove bay leaves and serve warm.

calories	fat	protein	carbs	fiber
356	28g	15g	12.1g	2.46g

PROTEIN PACKED KALE SALAD

Yield: 4 servings

Here is the king of all versatility. This delicious chopped kale dressed salad is ready to handle any protein you are craving . . . from sliced grilled beef to fried eggs. Make the dressing ahead of time and just keep it refrigerated until you need it.

2 garlic cloves, peeled and minced

3 tablespoons unsweetened almond milk

1 teaspoon cider vinegar

¼ teaspoon salt

¼ teaspoon black pepper

⅛ teaspoon paprika

½ cup olive oil

5 tablespoons grated Parmesan cheese

½ teaspoon sesame seeds

6 cups chopped kale

1 In the bowl of a food processor, combine the garlic, milk, vinegar, salt, pepper, and paprika.

2 With the motor running, slowly add the oil through the shoot until it's emulsified.

3 Add the Parmesan cheese and stir in the sesame seeds.

4 Refrigerate until ready to serve.

5 Toss kale and dressing in a large bowl.

6 Top with the protein of your choice.

PROTEIN OPTIONS:

1 pound grilled grass-fed steak

4 eggs, fried or poached

2 chicken breasts, grilled or roasted

2 avocados, peeled and sliced

4 slices nitrate-free bacon

Nutrition values for salad only.

calories	fat	protein	carbs	fiber
282	29.1g	3g	3.68g	0.96g

SPIRALIZED ZUCCHINI WITH BROWN BUTTER

Yield: 2 servings

Brown butter is different from ghee because it isn't strained. If possible, use a light colored skillet so you can easily see the butter brown to an amber color. You can double or triple the recipe.

2 tablespoons grass-fed butter, cut in pieces

2 tablespoons olive or avocado oil

2 garlic cloves, peeled and minced

¼ teaspoon onion salt

¼ teaspoon black pepper

⅛ teaspoon cayenne

2 zucchini, spiralized

1 tablespoon shredded Romano or Parmesan cheese

1 teaspoon chopped fresh chives

1 Place the butter in a large skillet over medium heat. Once it melts, it will crackle and pop. Stir constantly as the butter browns.

2 When it turns amber, remove from the heat and stir in the oil, garlic, salt, pepper, and cayenne.

3 Add the zucchini, tossing to coat, and return the pan to the stove. Cook 2 minutes.

4 Add the Romano or Parmesan cheese and chives.

5 Toss and serve warm.

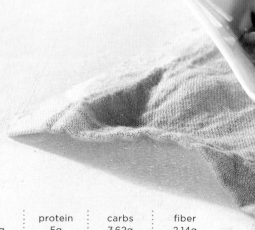

calories	fat	protein	carbs	fiber
288	27.6g	5g	7.62g	2.14g

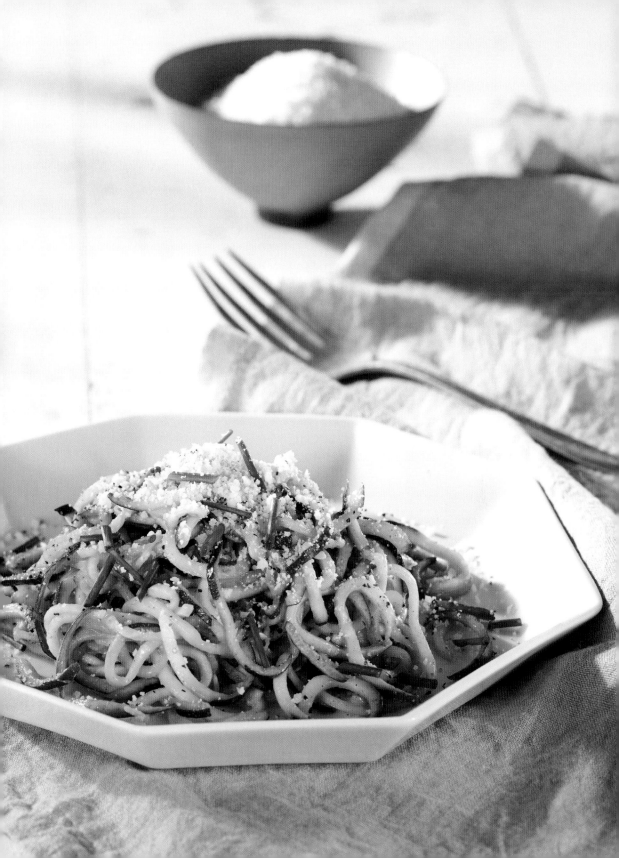

ALMOND GREEN BEAN SALAD

Yield: 6 servings

One slice of Turkey Meat Loaf (page 108) and a side of this chilled salad will make lunch something to look forward to all morning long. Substitute pecans or walnuts for the almonds if desired.

12 to 14 ounces (about 2 cups) trimmed green beans, halved crosswise

3 tablespoon almond oil

1 teaspoon cider vinegar

1 tablespoon avocado mayonnaise

⅛ teaspoon salt

⅛ teaspoon black pepper

1 small shallot, peeled and chopped

3 tablespoons slivered almonds

1 Place the green beans in a steamer basket over a pot of boiling water.

2 Cover and steam 5 to 6 minutes or until tender.

3 Transfer the steamer basket to a large container of ice water. Allow the beans to sit in the ice water for 2 minutes. Drain, pat dry with paper towels, and set aside.

4 Meanwhile, in a small bowl, whisk together the oil, vinegar, mayonnaise, salt, and pepper.

5 Place the cooled green beans and shallot in a serving bowl.

6 Toss gently with the dressing to evenly coat. Sprinkle the top with the almonds.

7 Cover and refrigerate at least 30 minutes before serving.

calories	fat	protein	carbs	fiber
118	11g	1.66g	4g	1.6g

CHOPPED SHRIMP SALAD WITH ITALIAN DRESSING

Yield: 2 servings

No knife is needed for this salad that is loaded with bite-sized goodness. The presentation is beautiful, and you can vary the ingredients as you wish.

DRESSING

¼ cup olive oil

2 tablespoons cider vinegar

1 small garlic clove, peeled and minced

1 tablespoon grated Romano or Parmesan cheese

½ teaspoon dried oregano

¼ teaspoon onion salt

⅛ teaspoon black pepper

SALAD

½ pound cooked shrimp, peeled, deveined, and chopped

1 heart of romaine lettuce, chopped

2 cups chopped radicchio

2 hard-boiled eggs, peeled and chopped

1 small cucumber, peeled and chopped

1 celery stalk, chopped

4 pimiento-stuffed olives, thinly sliced

1 green onion, sliced

1 In a jar with a tight-fitting lid, combine the oil, vinegar, garlic, cheese, oregano, salt, and pepper. Shake to emulsify, and set aside.

2 Place the shrimp, romaine, radicchio, eggs, cucumber, celery, olives, and onion in a large bowl, mixing well.

3 Cover and refrigerate.

4 When ready to serve, shake dressing, pour over salad, and toss. Serve chilled.

calories	fat	protein	carbs	fiber
602	40g	44.3g	18.1g	8.27g

GRILLED CHICKEN SALAD

Yield: 2 servings

*When you heat up the grill, always prepare extras
so you can pull this salad together in a snap.*

2 boneless chicken breasts

5 tablespoons olive oil, divided

½ teaspoon garlic salt

½ teaspoon black pepper

¼ teaspoon paprika

½ cucumber, peeled and chopped

2 tablespoons chopped black olives

1 green onion, chopped

1 small tomato, chopped

Baby spinach leaves

2 tablespoons cider vinegar

¼ cup shredded sharp Cheddar cheese

½ lime

1 Preheat the grill to medium-high.

2 Rub the chicken with 1 tablespoon oil and sprinkle evenly on both sides with the salt, pepper, and paprika.

3 Grill the chicken 6 minutes on each side or until no pink remains. Set aside to cool slightly before slicing.

4 Meanwhile, arrange the cucumber, olives, onions, and tomato over the spinach.

5 Whisk together 4 tablespoons oil and 2 tablespoons cider vinegar in a small bowl. Drizzle over spinach.

6 Top with the sliced chicken and then the Cheddar cheese. Squeeze the lime over the top and serve.

calories	fat	protein	carbs	fiber
695	46g	65.7g	7.35g	2.7g

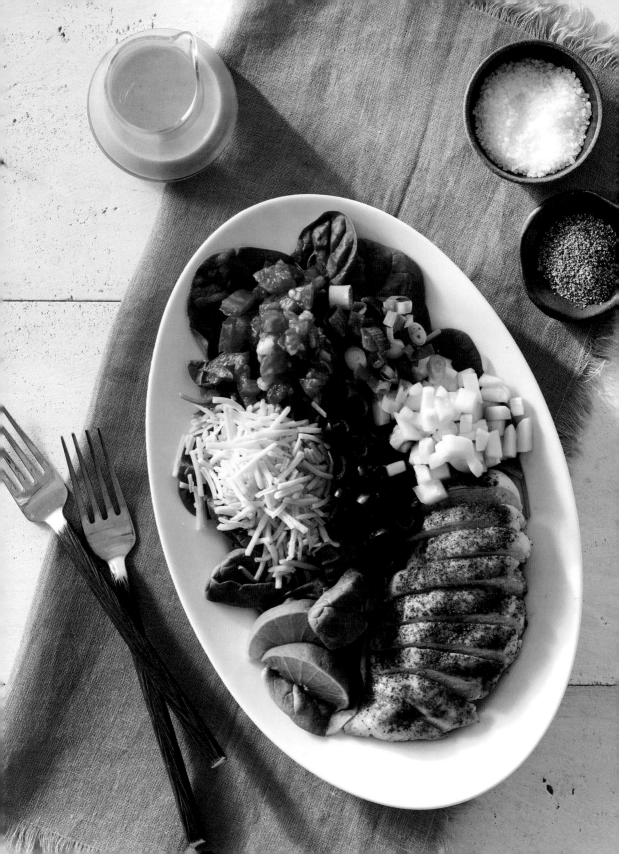

SHAVED ZUCCHINI SALAD

Yield: 4 servings

This is a warm salad for cool days. It pairs well with any leftover grilled meat or fish and is ready from start to finish in less than 15 minutes.

3 tablespoons avocado oil

1 large shallot, peeled and chopped

3 zucchini, trimmed and shaved into thin strips

1 Roma tomato, chopped

¼ teaspoon garlic salt

⅛ teaspoon black pepper

3 tablespoons julienned fresh basil

3 tablespoons grated Romano cheese

1 tablespoon lemon juice

1 Place the oil in a large skillet over medium-high heat.

2 When the skillet is hot, add the shallot and sauté 3 minutes, until translucent, stirring occasionally.

3 Add the zucchini, tomato, salt, and pepper to the skillet and cook an additional 5 minutes, stirring frequently.

4 Transfer to a serving bowl and toss with the basil, Romano cheese, and lemon juice. Serve warm.

calories	fat	protein	carbs	fiber
219	16.8g	9.3g	9.75g	2.4g

STIR-FRIED GREEN BEANS

Yield: 4 servings

*This versatile recipe can be used for any number of vegetables,
so feel free to substitute what you have on hand.
Two great options are bok choy or asparagus.*

1 pound fresh
green beans,
trimmed and cut in
2-inch pieces

4 tablespoons
grass-fed butter
(or ghee)

1 tablespoon fresh
ginger, chopped
and peeled

1 tablespoon
liquid aminos

4 tablespoons avocado
or olive oil

⅛ teaspoon
black pepper

1 tablespoon
sesame seeds

1 Place 1 cup of water in a large skillet over
high heat and bring to a boil.

2 Add the beans and return to a boil. Reduce
the heat to low, cover, and simmer 5 minutes.

3 Drain the beans into a colander and rinse
immediately under cold water. Set aside.

4 Place the butter in the same skillet and place
over high heat.

5 Add the beans, ginger, liquid aminos, oil,
and pepper. Cook 2 ½ minutes.

6 Remove from the heat and sprinkle with the
sesame seeds. Serve immediately.

calories	fat	protein	carbs	fiber
248	26.7g	1.17g	2.64g	0.99g

SHRIMP SKEWERS WITH WARM MUSHROOM SALAD

Yield: 2 servings

This is a terrific fall recipe to enjoy as the temperature shifts to sweater weather. Plan ahead to make sure the shrimp have plenty of time to marinate. It is equally delicious with grilled scallops.

½ pound large shrimp, peeled and deveined

4 tablespoons olive oil, divided

1 teaspoon dried oregano

1 teaspoon salt, divided

¼ teaspoon garlic powder

¼ teaspoon black pepper

2 tablespoons grass-fed butter (or ghee)

1 cup chopped mushrooms

¼ cup chopped toasted walnuts

2 cups baby arugula

1　Place the shrimp, 2 tablespoons olive oil, oregano, ½ teaspoon salt, garlic powder, and pepper in a zip-top bag and toss to coat. Refrigerate for 1 hour.

2　Place the butter in a medium skillet over medium-high heat.

3　When the skillet is hot, add the mushrooms and sprinkle with the remaining ½ teaspoon salt. Cook, stirring frequently, for 5 minutes.

4　Preheat the grill to medium.

5　Remove the shrimp from the marinade and thread on 2 skewers.

6　Grill 2 minutes and turn, grilling an additional 2 minutes. Set aside.

7　Stir the walnuts and remaining 2 tablespoons olive oil into the mushrooms and cook 2 minutes. Remove from heat.

8　Toss the arugula with the mushroom mixture for at least 1 minute to wilt the arugula slightly.

9　Serve with the shrimp.

calories	fat	protein	carbs	fiber
538	49.2g	21.2g	6.06g	2.16g

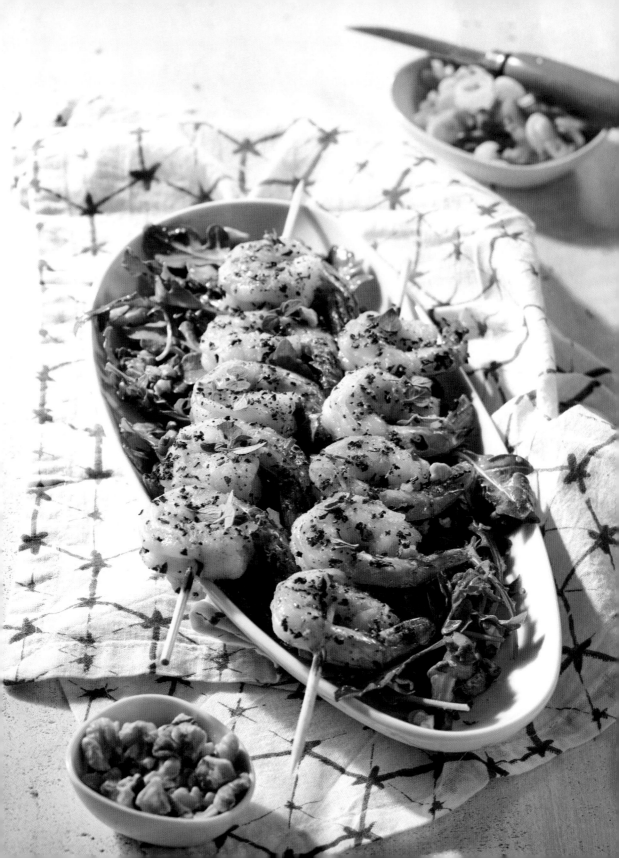

SALMON SALAD WRAPS

Yield: 2 servings

*One of the best values in the supermarket is canned wild salmon.
You can substitute tongal tuna or even lump crab meat for the salmon
in this recipe if desired. For the best flavor, make the salmon mixture
ahead and refrigerate before assembly.*

1 (7.5-ounce) can
wild salmon, drained

1 green onion,
chopped

4 tablespoons
avocado mayonnaise

¼ teaspoon
black pepper

4 large Boston or Bibb
lettuce leaves

4 cherry tomatoes,
halved

1   In a small mixing bowl, combine the salmon,
onion, mayonnaise, and pepper.

2   Arrange two lettuce leaves each on two serving
plates and evenly divide the salmon mixture
onto leaves.

3   Top with 2 tomatoes each and roll up, securing
with a toothpick if necessary. Serve immediately.

calories	fat	protein	carbs	fiber
380	28.4g	28.8g	2.52g	0.92g

CAULIFLOWER CRAB CAKES

Yield: 3 patties

*You'll be the envy of your workplace when caught eating this dish.
Serve over leafy greens and you're ready to face
the afternoon in the Keto Zone.*

1 cup lump crab meat

3 tablespoons avocado
or coconut oil

1 cup cooked &
mashed cauliflower

1 egg

3 tablespoons
minced celery

2 tablespoons
minced shallots

2 teaspoons chopped
fresh parsley

¼ teaspoon
white pepper

⅛ teaspoon cayenne

3 tablespoons
grass-fed butter
(or ghee)

1   In a medium mixing bowl, stir together the crab
meat, cauliflower, egg, celery, shallots, parsley,
pepper, cayenne, and oil. Form into 3 patties
and place on a waxed paper-lined plate.

2   Cover with plastic wrap and refrigerate at least
1 hour.

3   Place the butter in a large skillet over
medium-high heat.

4   Add the patties and brown 3 minutes on each
side. Flip only once.

5   Serve warm, or cool completely and serve at
room temperature.

calories	fat	protein	carbs	fiber
303	28g	11g	3g	1.12g

TURKEY MEAT LOAF

Yield: 6 servings

One of the few meat dishes that always seems to taste better the following day is meat loaf. Plan ahead in order to have this comfort food at lunch for a couple of days. It freezes very well. Serve with Almond Green Bean Salad (page 90).

1 pound ground turkey

½ pound
  hot turkey sausage

1 small onion, peeled
  and minced

2 eggs

6 tablespoons
  avocado oil

½ teaspoon garlic salt

¼ teaspoon
  black pepper

1 Preheat the oven to 350 degrees. Lightly grease a loaf pan with olive oil cooking spray and set aside.

2 In a large mixing bowl, use your hands to combine the ground turkey, turkey sausage, onion, eggs, oil, salt, and pepper.

3 Transfer the turkey mixture to the prepared loaf pan and bake 50 minutes or until an instant-read thermometer reads 170 degrees in the center.

4 Allow to rest at least 10 minutes or cool completely before slicing.

5 Drizzle with Tangy BBQ sauce (page 44), if desired.

calories	fat	protein	carbs	fiber
343	28.3g	20.5g	1.92g	0.14g

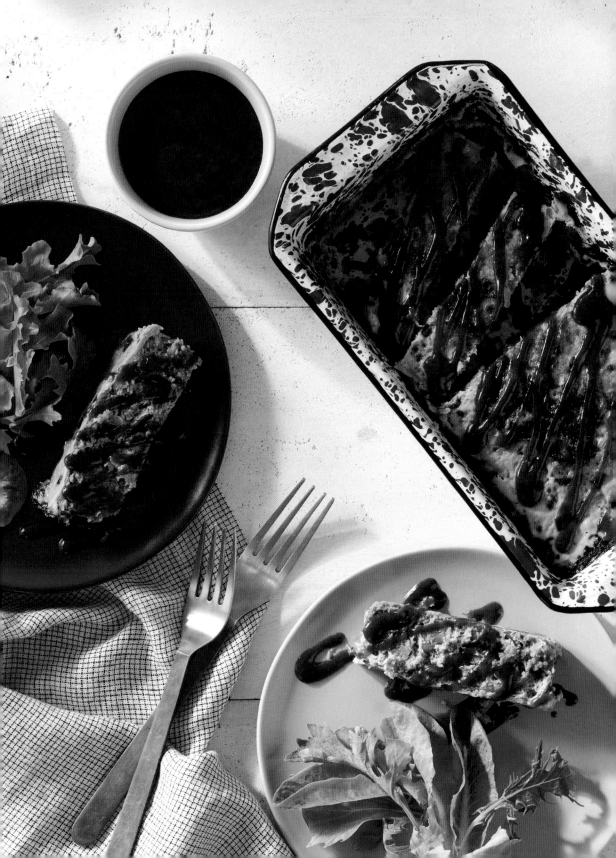

BOK CHOY & TILAPIA FISH PACKETS

Yield: 4 servings

Search for baby bok choy for this recipe, which is just the perfect size to enhance the flavor. The smaller leaves are more tender than the larger ones and have a milder taste. Fresh ginger is just the spark it needs.

4 bunches of baby bok choy, trimmed and cut in half lengthwise

1 large shallot, peeled and cut in 4 pieces

2 teaspoons fresh ginger, peeled and grated

2 teaspoons liquid aminos

4 tablespoons avocado oil

1 teaspoon cider vinegar

4 tablespoons grass-fed butter (or ghee), divided

4 wild tilapia fillets

¼ teaspoon garlic salt

¼ teaspoon black pepper

1 Preheat the oven to 450 degrees.

2 Cut parchment paper into four 20x13-inch rectangles. Spray one side of each with olive oil cooking spray.

3 Evenly divide the bok choy, shallot, and ginger between the parchment paper pieces.

4 Drizzle evenly with the liquid aminos, oil, and vinegar and top with the fish fillets. Place 1 tablespoon butter on top of each fish fillet.

5 Sprinkle with the salt and pepper.

6 Fold the parchment paper over the tilapia to make a packet and arrange on a large baking pan. Bake 12 minutes and transfer to a serving plate.

7 Carefully open each packet, allowing steam to escape. Serve immediately.

calories	fat	protein	carbs	fiber
380	28g	27.4g	8.33g	2.8g

TURKEY TENDERLOIN KABOBS

Yield: 3 servings

No need to fire up the grill because the oven broiler takes care of this quick lunch! You will need 3 skewers for this recipe.

1 pound turkey tenderloins, cut in large cubes

¼ cup liquid aminos

1 tablespoon lime juice

1 tablespoon olive oil

½ teaspoon garlic salt

¼ teaspoon black pepper

1 onion, peeled, quartered, and separated into slices

1 zucchini, trimmed and cut in thick chunks

1 Place the turkey in a large zip-top bag.

2 In a jar with a tight-fitting lid, combine the liquid aminos, lime juice, oil, salt, and pepper. Shake to emulsify and pour over the turkey. Seal and refrigerate for at least 2 hours.

3 Preheat the broiler and lightly grease a roasting rack with olive oil cooking spray and set over a rimmed baking sheet.

4 Thread the turkey pieces alternately with the onion and zucchini onto 3 skewers.

5 Place on the rack and broil 4 minutes. Turn the kabobs twice more and broil 3 to 4 minutes with each turn until the turkey is done and no pink remains. Serve warm. Use Tzatiki (page 45) or Salsa Verde (page 51) as a dipping sauce with the kabobs, if desired.

OPTION: Substitute grass-fed beef for turkey.

calories	fat	protein	carbs	fiber
306	15.4g	39.3g	8.04g	1.37g

SPICY LAMB MEATBALLS
WITH TZATZIKI

Yield: 3 servings

*This might quickly become your favorite make-ahead lunch item.
The spices in these incredible meatballs give them a Middle Eastern flair.
You can also use a beef and lamb mixture if desired. Make the sauce
at least the day before so the flavors have a chance to meld.*

TZATZIKI SAUCE

1 medium cucumber,
peeled, seeded, and
grated

½ teaspoon salt

1 cup sour cream

1 large garlic clove,
peeled and minced

1 tablespoon
lemon juice

3 tablespoons olive oil

¼ teaspoon
white pepper

1 tablespoon chopped
fresh dill

1 Line a colander with a paper towel or
cheesecloth. Place the cucumber in the
colander and sprinkle with the salt. Let stand
at room temperature 30 minutes.

2 Squeeze to remove any excess moisture and
transfer to a medium mixing bowl.

3 Add the sour cream, garlic, lemon juice,
oil, pepper, and dill. Stir well, cover, and
refrigerate.

calories	fat	protein	carbs	fiber
290	28.5g	2.69g	8.15g	0.63g

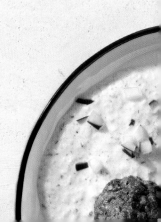

MEATBALLS

½ onion, peeled

3 garlic cloves, peeled

2 tablespoons chopped fresh parsley

1 teaspoon fresh oregano, chopped

½ teaspoon crushed red pepper

1 pound ground grass-fed lamb

1 teaspoon ground cumin

½ heaping teaspoon ground coriander

1 teaspoon salt

1 Preheat the oven to 425 degrees.

2 Place the onion, garlic, parsley, oregano, and crushed red pepper in the bowl of a food processor, and pulse until very finely chopped.

3 Transfer to a large mixing bowl and add the lamb, cumin, coriander, and salt.

4 Using your hands, mix well. Form into 1-inch meatballs and place on a baking sheet lined with parchment paper, making sure the meatballs don't touch.

5 Bake meatballs 9 to 11 minutes until slightly browned and cooked through.

6 Remove and cool at least 5 minutes before serving. Or cool completely and serve at room temperature.

calories	fat	protein	carbs	fiber
443	35.6g	25.6g	3.74g	.88g

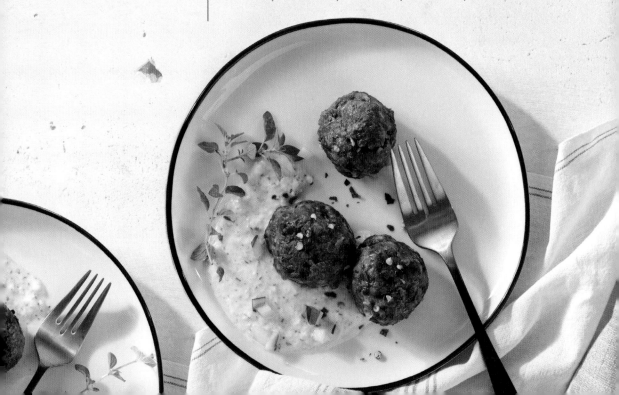

SESAME TURKEY

Yield: 3 servings

One of the fastest ways to prepare lunch is to stir-fry. A wok is best but if you don't have one, use a large bowl-shaped skillet. The key is high heat! Serve with Stir-Fried Green Beans (page 95).

3 tablespoons ghee

1 pound turkey tenderloins, cut in bite-sized pieces

1 tablespoon fresh ginger, peeled and finely minced

3 tablespoons avocado oil

½ teaspoon garlic salt

¼ teaspoon black pepper

1 tablespoon sesame seeds

1 Place the ghee in a wok over high heat.

2 When it's hot, add the turkey and ginger. Stir-fry 5 minutes, stirring constantly, until the turkey is no longer pink.

3 Add the oil and sprinkle with the salt, pepper, and sesame seeds. Cook 1 minute longer, stirring constantly. Serve warm.

calories	fat	protein	carbs	fiber
492	38.8g	33.6g	1.18g	0.44g

CHICKEN & GREEN BEAN LETTUCE WRAPS

Yield: 3 servings

This is a perfect make-ahead lunch meal. Prepare the filling the night before and simply reheat or serve at room temperature.

2 (6-ounce) boneless chicken breasts, sliced in thin strips

½ cup green beans, cut in ⅓-inch pieces

1 small celery stalk, chopped

2 small garlic cloves, peeled and minced

1½ teaspoons cider vinegar

1½ teaspoons liquid aminos

3 tablespoons grass-fed butter (or ghee)

4 tablespoons olive or avocado oil, divided

½ teaspoon fresh ginger, peeled and grated

¼ teaspoon lime zest

¼ teaspoon black pepper

6 large romaine lettuce leaves

1 In a medium mixing bowl, stir together the chicken, green beans, celery, garlic, vinegar, liquid aminos, 3 tablespoons oil, ginger, lime zest, and pepper. Cover and refrigerate for 1 hour.

2 Place the butter in a large skillet over medium-high heat.

3 When the skillet is hot, add the chicken mixture and sauté for 10 minutes or until the chicken is cooked through.

4 Remove from the heat, add 1 tablespoon oil, and let stand 5 minutes. If making ahead, put the filling in an airtight container and refrigerate until ready to assemble.

5 Place a large spoonful of the chicken mixture in the center of each lettuce leaf and roll it like a burrito. Serve immediately.

calories	fat	protein	carbs	fiber
386	35.8g	13.7g	4.15g	1.81g

LOW & SLOW CHICKEN THIGHS

Yield: 6 servings

All this recipe requires is some preplanning. Get it started early in the morning and by lunchtime, you've got a meal that can be served a number of different ways. It is great served with Creamed Spinach (page 152), or you can wrap it in lettuce leaves, or chill it and pile it on microgreens. There are endless possibilities!

2 cups chicken bone broth (page 38)

½ cup grass-fed butter

½ teaspoon garlic salt

½ teaspoon onion salt

½ teaspoon black pepper

½ teaspoon cayenne

2 pounds boneless chicken thighs

1   Place the chicken broth and butter in a medium (4-quart) slow cooker.

2   In a small bowl, mix together the garlic salt, onion salt, pepper, and cayenne.

3   Rub the salt mixture all over the chicken thighs and carefully place them in the broth. Cover and cook on low for 4½ to 5 hours.

4   Serve warm, at room temperature, or chilled.

NOTE: If desired, shred the chicken after removing from the cooking liquid.

calories	fat	protein	carbs	fiber
463	38.4g	27.2g	3.04g	0.09g

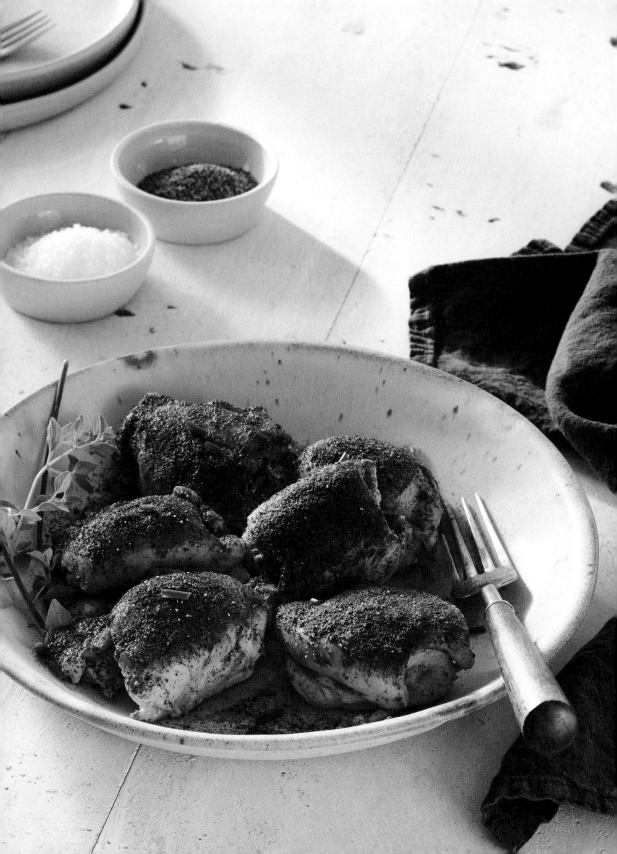

BAKED BUFFALO CHICKEN WINGS

yields: 4 servings

These wings are excellent as a game day snack or lunchtime meal.
Served with avocado mayonnaise dip and you'll be licking your fingers clean!

WINGS:

16 chicken wings
(if frozen, thawed)

2 tablespoons avocado
or olive oil

4 tablespoons
grass-fed butter
(or ghee)

¼ cup hot sauce

1 teaspoon garlic,
minced

¼ teaspoon paprika

½ teaspoon salt

¼ teaspoon
black pepper

DIPPING SAUCE:

¼ cup avocado
mayonnaise

¼ cup sour cream

1 teaspoon cayenne

3 scallions, finely
chopped

WINGS:

1 Preheat the oven to 375 degrees. Place a wire rack inside a large baking dish.

2 Rub oil over chicken wings and evenly spread wings on wire rack. Sprinkle with salt and pepper.

3 Bake wings for about 45 minutes or until wings are getting crispy on edges.

4 While wings bake, add 1 tablespoon butter to a saucepan to melt over medium heat. Once butter is melted, add garlic, and cook for 1 minute.

5 Reduce heat to low, add hot sauce, remaining butter, and paprika, and mix together.

6 Once butter has melted and sauce is hot, remove from heat.

7 Remove wings from oven and toss in sauce.

8 Serve warm with dipping sauce.

DIPPING SAUCE:

1 Whisk together ingredients until blended smooth.

2 Serve with baked chicken wings.

3 Store leftovers in airtight container in the refrigerator.

calories	fat	protein	carbs	fiber
1081	84g	75.8g	1.86g	0.48g

CREAMY SOUTHERN STYLE CHICKEN SALAD

Yields: 4 servings

Going Keto doesn't mean you need to give up all of your favorite comfort foods. Toss together this chicken salad and you can stay in the Keto Zone and fill a craving all at the same time.

2 organic pastured boneless chicken breast

2 tablespoons grass-fed butter, softened

2 large eggs, hard-boiled (see page 58)

1 cup avocado mayonnaise

2 tablespoons red onion, diced

1 celery stalk, diced

1 tablespoon dill pickle, chopped

¼ teaspoon chili powder

1 teaspoon salt

1 teaspoon black pepper

Pinch of cilantro as garnish (optional)

1 Preheat oven to 400 degrees. Place chicken on a baking dish.

2 Rub softened butter all over chicken breasts and season with ½ teaspoon salt, and ½ teaspoon pepper. Place chicken breasts in a roasting pan, skin side up.

3 Roast chicken for 15 minutes, then flip chicken and bake another 10–12 minutes, or until chicken is no longer pink.

4 In a medium bowl, combine chicken, onion, celery, and egg.

5 In a small bowl, combine mayonnaise, pickle, chili powder, ½ teaspoon salt, and ½ teaspoon pepper. Mix well.

6 Add mayonnaise mixture to bowl with chicken and stir with a fork until well blended.

7 Garnish with fresh cilantro if desired.

8 Use immediately or refrigerate until chilled and serve with large leaf lettuce. Store in refrigerator.

calories	fat	protein	carbs	fiber
270	19g	21.5g	1.4g	0.41g

STEAMED VEGETABLES

Yield: 2 servings

Steaming vegetables is much better than boiling—the nutrients are preserved! This quick recipe is great if you're in a hurry or looking to add some green to your meat dish.

3 to 4 cups vegetables of your choice, washed and cut in equal sizes

1 steamer basket

2 to 3 small sprigs of fresh herbs, such as thyme or rosemary (optional)

2 tablespoons grass-fed butter

2 tablespoons avocado oil

1 Bring at least 2 inches of water in a Dutch oven to a boil over medium-high heat.

2 Place the vegetables in the steamer basket.

3 If desired, place a few small sprigs of fresh herbs in the water.

4 Reduce the heat to low and insert the steamer basket into the Dutch oven. Cover and simmer according to the guide here or until the vegetables are easily pierced with a paring knife in their thickest part.

5 Drain and add 2 tablespoons grass-fed butter and 2 tablespoons avocado oil. Toss to coat and butter melts or oil is warmed.

Nutrition varies by vegetable.
See pages 23–24 for net carb amounts.

VEGETABLE STEAMING TIMES

Asparagus spears	5 to 6 minutes
Broccoli florets	4 to 5 minutes
Broccoli spears	5 to 7 minutes
Brussels sprouts	8 to 9 minutes
Cauliflower	7 to 9 minutes
Sugar Snap or Snow peas	3 to 5 minutes
Green beans	8 minutes
Kale, trimmed	4 to 7 minutes
Squash, winter	15 to 20 minutes
Squash, summer	4 to 5 minutes

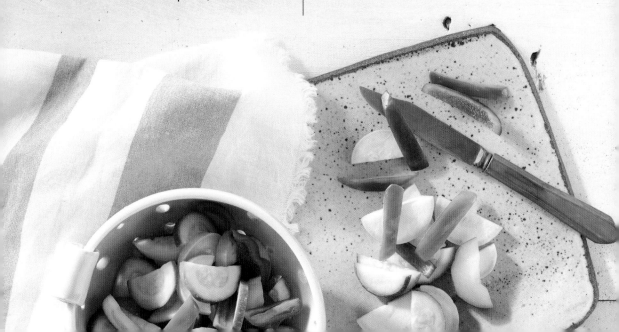

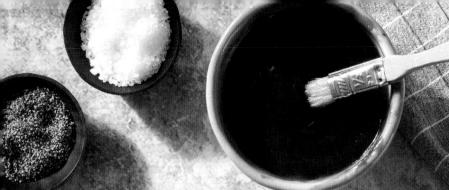

DINNER RECIPES

DINNER

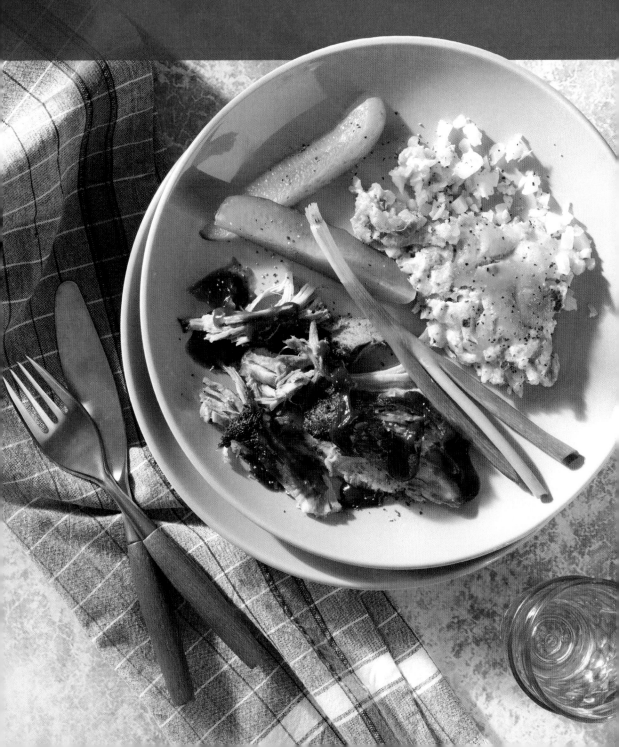

BASIL BAKED TILAPIA

Yield: 3 servings

*A pesto-like topping makes this recipe a favorite. As with all fish,
watch it carefully to make sure not to overcook.*

3 (3-ounce)
tilapia fillets

½ cup fresh basil,
chopped

3 tablespoons olive oil

1 large garlic clove,
peeled and minced

1½ teaspoons
lemon juice

¼ teaspoon salt

¼ teaspoon
black pepper

3 tablespoons
grass-fed butter
(or ghee), divided

½ lemon, cut in small
wedges

1 Preheat the oven to 350 degrees.

2 Lightly grease an 11x9-inch baking dish with
olive oil cooking spray and add the tilapia fillets.

3 In a small bowl, stir together the basil, oil,
garlic, lemon juice, salt, and pepper.

4 Spoon evenly over the fillets.

5 Place 1 tablespoon butter over each filet.

6 Bake 15 minutes or until the fish flakes easily
with a fork. Serve warm with the lemon wedges.

calories	fat	protein	carbs	fiber
337	27g	23.6g	1.08g	0.16g

GRILLED LEMON PEPPER SALMON

Yield: 2 servings

Look for wild salmon when it goes on sale and stock extra for the freezer. This citrus enhanced fillet goes well with practically any side dish.

2 (6-ounce) wild salmon fillets

3 tablespoons olive oil

1 tablespoon lemon juice

½ teaspoon black pepper

1 teaspoon minced garlic, divided

2 tablespoons grass-fed butter (or ghee), divided

2 lemon wedges

1 Place the salmon in a shallow dish and set aside.

2 In a jar with a tight-fitting lid, combine the oil, lemon juice, and pepper. Shake to emulsify and pour over the salmon. Let stand at room temperature 20 minutes, turning after 10 minutes.

3 Preheat the grill to medium-high.

4 Place the salmon on the hottest part of the grill and sear for 2 minutes on each side.

5 Move the salmon to indirect heat and add ½ teaspoon garlic and 1 tablespoon butter to each fillet.

6 Grill 6 to 8 minutes or to the desired degree of doneness.

7 Serve warm with the lemon wedges.

calories	fat	protein	carbs	fiber
850	56.9g	79g	1.77g	0.22g

LEMON & GARLIC BAKED FISH

Yield: 2 servings

*This delicious recipe can be used for preparing any flaky fish.
It is particularly nice with salmon, haddock, cod, or halibut.*

2 (6-ounce) fish fillets

2 tablespoons olive oil

½ lemon

2 small garlic cloves,
peeled and minced

¼ teaspoon salt

¼ teaspoon
black pepper

¼ teaspoon
crushed red pepper

2 tablespoons
grass-fed butter
(or ghee), divided

1 teaspoon chopped
fresh chives

1 Preheat the oven to 400 degrees.

2 Place the oil in an 8x8-inch casserole dish and place the fillets on top. Squeeze the lemon over the fillets and sprinkle evenly with the garlic, salt, pepper, and crushed red pepper.

3 Top each fillet with 1 tablespoon of butter.

4 Cover with foil and bake 12 minutes or until the fish flakes easily with a fork. Top with the chives and serve warm.

calories	fat	protein	carbs	fiber
495	36.7g	38.2g	2.16g	0.25g

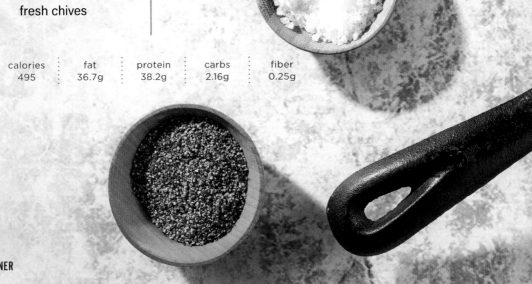

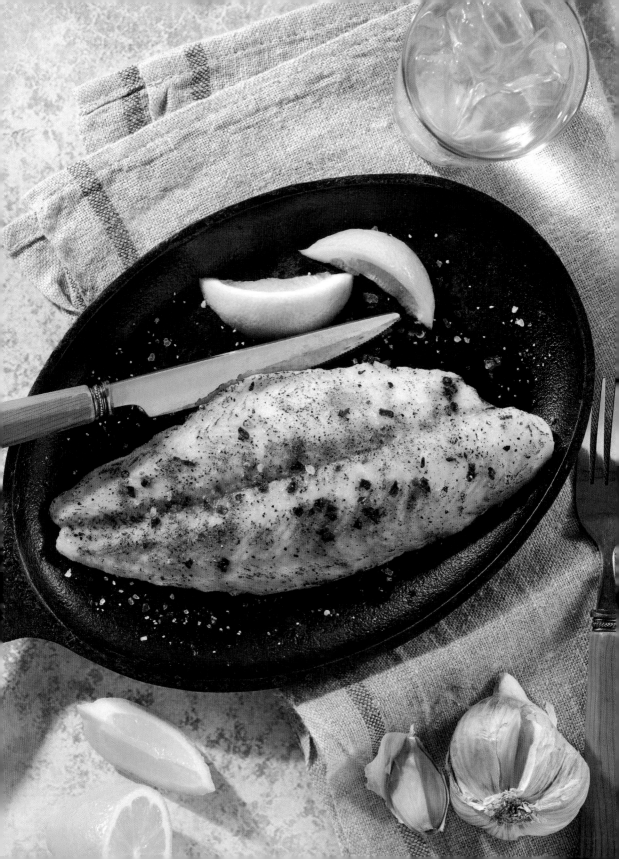

FLOUNDER THYME

Yield: 3 servings

The delicate flavor and fine texture of flounder make it the perfect fish for showcasing fresh thyme. Any leftovers are excellent the following day for lunch.

3 tablespoons avocado oil

3 sprigs fresh thyme, finely chopped

1 small garlic clove, peeled and minced

¼ teaspoon onion salt

¼ teaspoon black pepper

⅛ teaspoon paprika

Pinch of cayenne

1½ pounds flounder fillets

3 tablespoons grass-fed butter (or ghee), divided

½ cup finely chopped broccoli

½ lemon

1 Preheat the oven to 350 degrees.

2 Place the oil in the bottom of a 13x9-inch baking dish and set aside.

3 In a small bowl, combine the thyme, garlic, salt, pepper, paprika, and cayenne. Rub over the flounder and place in the prepared baking dish.

4 Add 1 tablespoon of butter to each flounder fillet and top with the broccoli.

5 Bake for 15 minutes or until the fish flakes easily with a fork. Squeeze the lemon over the baked fish before serving it hot.

calories	fat	protein	carbs	fiber
368	29.3g	24.2g	2.18g	0.58g

COCONUT FISH FILLETS

Yield: 4 servings

Hints of coconut allow naturally sweet fish fillets to have just the right amount of flavor. They bake to a crispy goodness and are served with tartar sauce (page 41).

4 tablespoons melted coconut oil, divided

2 tablespoons flax meal

2 tablespoons coconut flour

2 tablespoons finely grated Parmesan cheese

1 teaspoon onion salt, divided

¼ teaspoon black pepper

¼ teaspoon paprika

1 egg

1 tablespoon coconut milk

4 tilapia fillets

1 Prepare the tartar sauce from page 41, cover, and refrigerate until ready to serve with hot fish.

2 Preheat the oven to 400 degrees. Line a baking sheet with parchment paper and brush with 2 tablespoons coconut oil.

3 In a large zip-top bag, add the flax meal, flour, Parmesan cheese, ½ teaspoon salt, pepper, and paprika. Set aside.

4 In a shallow container, whisk together the egg and coconut milk.

5 Dip each fish fillet into the egg mixture, then place in the bag and shake to coat.

6 Place the fillets on the prepared baking sheet.

7 Drizzle with 2 tablespoons coconut oil and bake for 22 to 25 minutes or until golden brown.

8 Serve immediately with tartar sauce.

calories	fat	protein	carbs	fiber
304	20.2g	26.8g	3.83g	2.38g

WILTED BABY SPINACH
WITH PAN-SEARED SALMON

Yield: 2 servings

*What a combination! It looks company worthy and tastes like you
spent a lot more time than is required to get it on the table.
Prepare the spinach first, then the salmon. It can easily be doubled.*

2 (6-ounce)
wild salmon fillets

1 teaspoon salt,
divided

3 tablespoons
grass-fed butter
(or ghee), divided

1 garlic clove, peeled
and minced

Pinch of crushed
red pepper

1 small head escarole,
chopped

2 cups baby spinach

¼ teaspoon
lemon zest

2 tablespoons
avocado oil, divided

1 Season the salmon with ½ teaspoon salt and
set aside.

2 Place 2 tablespoons butter in a large skillet
over high heat.

3 Add the garlic and crushed red pepper, and
cook 30 seconds.

4 Turn heat down to medium and stir in the
escarole and remaining ½ teaspoon salt. Cook,
stirring often, until the escarole is wilted, about
2 minutes.

5 Turn off the heat and add the spinach and
lemon zest. Set aside.

6 Place 1 tablespoon of oil and 1 tablespoon of
butter in a medium skillet over medium-high
heat.

7 When the skillet is hot, add the salmon, flesh-
side down. Cook 4 minutes without touching.
Flip the fillets and cook an additional 3 minutes
on the other side or until the salmon is cooked
through.

8 Toss the spinach mixture with the remaining
1 tablespoon of oil and use as a base for the
salmon.

calories	fat	protein	carbs	fiber
888	56.6g	83g	10.3g	8.7g

DILL GRILLED SALMON

Yield: 2 servings

*Feathery fresh dill adds just the right punch in flavor for wild salmon steaks.
Go ahead and double the recipe if you can . . . it's that good!*

2 tablespoons olive oil

1 tablespoon
tarragon vinegar

1 tablespoon chopped
fresh dill

½ teaspoon
garlic powder

¼ teaspoon
white pepper

Juice of 1 lemon

2 (4-ounce)
salmon fillets

2 tablespoons
grass-fed butter
(or ghee), divided

1 In a small mixing bowl, combine the oil, vinegar, dill, garlic powder, pepper, and lemon juice.

2 Pour over the salmon, cover, and refrigerate at least 1 hour, turning after 30 minutes.

3 Preheat the grill to medium-high.

4 Place 1 tablespoon of butter over each fillet.

5 Cook 3 to 5 minutes on each side or until the salmon is done. Serve warm.

calories	fat	protein	carbs	fiber
796	50.3g	79.2g	2.9g	0.34g

GRILLED PROSCIUTTO WRAPPED SCALLOPS

Yield: 4 servings

All you need to make this meal complete is a special occasion.
Watch the scallops carefully so they don't overcook.
You will need 4 skewers for this recipe.

6 prosciutto slices

12 large scallops

3 tablespoons +
1 teaspoon olive oil,
divided

2 lemons, cut in half

3 tablespoons
grass-fed butter
(or ghee), melted

6 cups baby arugula

¼ teaspoon garlic salt

¼ teaspoon
black pepper

3 tablespoons
toasted pine nuts

1 Preheat the grill to medium-high.

2 Using kitchen shears, cut each prosciutto slice
in half lengthwise. Roll the prosciutto around
the edges of the scallops, securing on skewers.
Brush all sides with 1 tablespoon oil. Brush the
cut sides of the lemons with 1 teaspoon oil.

3 Place the skewers and lemon halves (cut side
down) on the hot grill. Turn the scallops after
2 or 3 minutes and grill an additional
2 minutes. Remove the skewers and lemons
from the grill. Drizzle the melted butter over
the scallop skewers.

4 Carefully remove the scallops from the skewers
and immediately plate on top of individual
servings of baby arugula.

5 Sprinkle evenly with the salt, pepper, and
toasted pine nuts. Serve each plate with
a charred lemon half.

calories	fat	protein	carbs	fiber
441	39.5g	15.1g	14.3g	6.1g

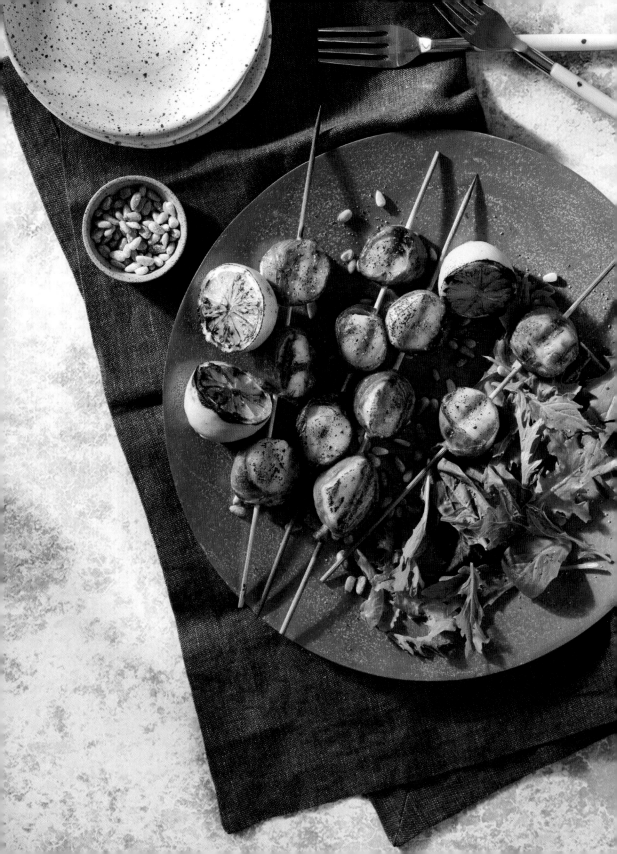

HERB ROASTED CHICKEN

Yield: 5 servings

This simple, rustic dish is a beautiful centerpiece for a nice dinner. The key is not to baste or open the oven door during roasting. Position the roasting pan so you can readily view the meat thermometer through the oven window.

1 (3 ½ pound)
  whole chicken
  thawed, if frozen,
  with neck and
  giblets removed

1 lemon

6 tablespoons
  grass-fed butter
  (or ghee), softened

1 teaspoon fresh basil,
  chopped

1 teaspoon fresh
  chives, chopped

1 teaspoon fresh
  oregano, chopped

1 teaspoon fresh
  parsley, chopped

1 teaspoon fresh
  thyme, chopped

½ teaspoon garlic salt

¼ teaspoon
  black pepper

1. Preheat the oven to 375 degrees.

2. Lightly grease the rack of a roasting pan with olive oil cooking spray and place the chicken breast side up on rack.

3. Pierce the lemon several times with an ice pick or knife tip and insert into the cavity of the chicken.

4. Truss the chicken legs and lift the wing tips over the back of the chicken, tucking underneath.

5. In a small bowl, stir together the butter, basil, chives, oregano, parsley, thyme, salt, and pepper.

6. Brush the chicken with all of the butter mixture.

7. Insert a meat thermometer into a thigh, making sure it doesn't touch the bone. Roast for 80 minutes or until the thermometer registers 165 degrees. Let the chicken rest 10 minutes before slicing and serving warm.

VARIATION:

1. Omit the herb and butter mixture and substitute a half recipe of Herbed Goat Cheese (page 180).

2. Loosen the chicken skin without tearing any holes and carefully insert the softened goat cheese underneath the skin and on top of the meat.

3. Using your fingers, massage the cheese so that it covers the meat. Insert the meat thermometer and roast as directed.

calories	fat	protein	carbs	fiber
771	60.6g	52.1g	3g	1.2g

LEMON BASIL CHICKEN

Yield: 4 servings

The ingredient list is short but the flavor is huge!
You can substitute chicken breasts for the thighs if desired.

3 tablespoons
lemon juice

2 tablespoons fresh
basil, chopped

½ teaspoon garlic salt

½ teaspoon
black pepper

¼ cup olive oil

4 chicken thighs

1 Place the lemon juice, basil, salt, and pepper in a food processer and process for 5 seconds, or until combined. Slowly add the oil through the shoot and continue to process until blended.

2 Reserve half of the basil mixture and pour the remainder into a large ziplock bag and add chicken. Seal and refrigerate for 30 minutes.

3 Preheat the grill to medium.

4 Grill the chicken 20 to 30 minutes, basting with the reserved marinade. Continue grilling until no pink remains and an instant-read thermometer registers 170 degrees. Serve warm.

calories	fat	protein	carbs	fiber
599	53.4g	30.1g	1.01g	0.13g

GRILLED CHICKEN WITH AVOCADO CITRUS CREAM

Yield: 6 servings

This sauce is delicate but flavorful and excellent for dinner with friends. It is beautiful with grilled chicken, but an equally nice complement to fish and shellfish.

6 boneless chicken breast halves

1 teaspoon garlic salt, divided

½ teaspoon black pepper, divided

3 tablespoons grass-fed butter, divided

3 garlic cloves, peeled and minced

1 cup heavy whipping cream, at room temperature

3 tablespoons lime juice

1 teaspoon lime zest

1 avocado, peeled, pitted, and mashed

Lime wedges

1 Preheat the grill to medium-high.

2 Sprinkle the chicken with ½ teaspoon salt and ¼ teaspoon pepper. Set aside.

3 Place 1 tablespoon butter in a small saucepan over medium heat.

4 Add the garlic and sauté until soft, about a minutes.

5 Reduce the heat to low and slowly stir in the cream.

6 Add the lime juice and zest.

7 Whisk in the avocado until smooth. Season with the remaining ½ teaspoon salt and ¼ teaspoon pepper.

8 Cover and remove from the heat.

9 Melt the remaining 2 tablespoons butter and brush the chicken breasts on both sides.

10 Grill, turning once, for 6 to 8 minutes on each side or until no pink remains.

11 Serve warm with the Avocado Citrus Cream sauce and garnish plates with lime wedges.

calories	fat	protein	carbs	fiber
545	41.1g	38.3g	5.83g	2.39g

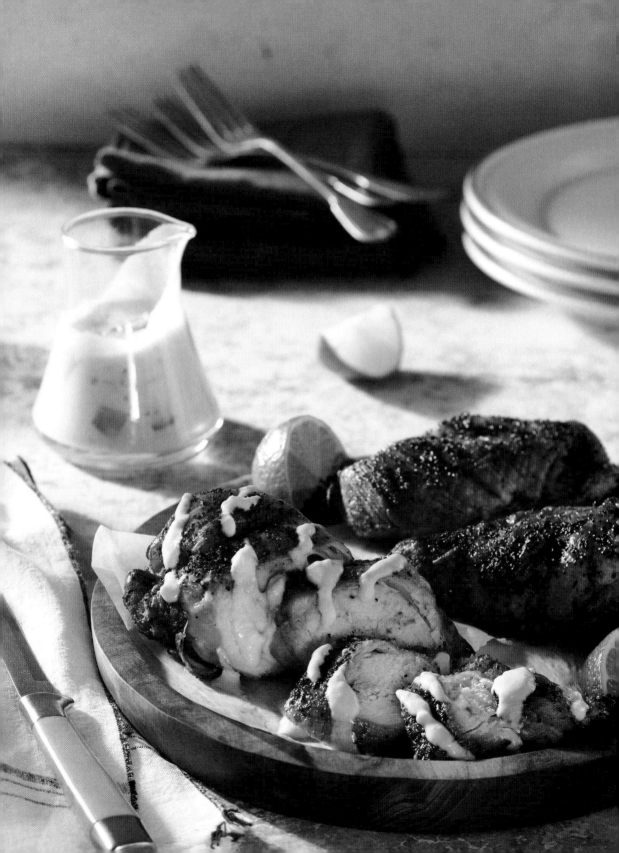

HOT LIME LEG QUARTERS

Yield: 3 servings

Using seeded jalapeño peppers cuts some of the heat,
but still gives this chicken an exclamation mark!
If you want it a bit milder, decrease the number of peppers.

4 jalapeño peppers, sliced in half with seeds and membranes removed

1 green onion, cut in large pieces

3 tablespoons lime juice

2 tablespoons cider vinegar

3 tablespoons avocado mayonnaise (or sour cream)

1 teaspoon dried basil

1 teaspoon dried thyme

1 teaspoon mustard seeds

½ teaspoon garlic salt

½ teaspoon black pepper

3 chicken leg quarters

1   Place the peppers, onion, lime juice, vinegar, mayonnaise, basil, thyme, mustard seeds, salt, and pepper in the bowl of a food processor and blend until smooth.

2   Place the chicken in a shallow baking dish and spread the pepper mixture all over. Refrigerate uncovered for at least 2 hours.

3   Preheat the grill to medium.

4   Grill for 30 to 40 minutes or until a meat thermometer registers 170 degrees when inserted in the thickest part of the chicken.

5   Let rest at least 10 minutes before serving warm.

NOTE: Top with Salsa Verde (page 51) for added flavor.

calories	fat	protein	carbs	fiber
761	55.9g	56.9g	4.17g	1.05g

SEARED CHICKEN THIGHS

Yield: 2 servings

*Placing chicken thighs skin down in a hot pan produces
a crispy skin that will satisfy your need for crunch.
Serve hot to take advantage of the crackly texture.*

2 tablespoons
avocado oil

2 chicken thighs

½ teaspoon onion salt

¼ teaspoon
black pepper

⅛ teaspoon paprika

1 Remove the chicken from the refrigerator
15 minutes before preparing.

2 Place the oil in a medium oven-proof skillet
over medium-high heat.

3 Sprinkle the chicken evenly with the salt,
pepper, and paprika. Place the chicken in the
hot oil with the skin side down. Cook without
touching for 8 minutes.

4 Meanwhile, preheat the oven to 400 degrees.

5 Turn the chicken and cook an additional
3 to 5 minutes. Remove the skillet from the
stove, flip the thighs so the skin side is up, and
bake 12 minutes or until the chicken is no longer
pink or registers 170 degrees on an instant read
thermometer.

6 Let rest 5 minutes before serving hot.

calories	fat	protein	carbs	fiber
460	37.9g	30.1g	0.27g	0.12g

STUFFED CHICKEN CUTLETS

Yield: 4 servings

The cheese and prosciutto stuffing is a nice surprise for this grilled dinner dish. Leftovers can be sliced and served as snacks. You will need 4 skewers for this recipe.

4 pastured chicken cutlets

½ teaspoon garlic salt

¼ teaspoon black pepper

¼ teaspoon dried oregano

¼ teaspoon crushed red pepper

4 slices provolone cheese

4 slices prosciutto

3 tablespoons chopped fresh parsley, divided

2 tablespoons avocado oil

½ lemon

1 Preheat the grill to medium-high.

2 Place each chicken cutlet between 2 large pieces of plastic wrap. Using a meat mallet or heavy pan, pound evenly to ½ inch thickness.

3 Lay the chicken on a waxed paper-lined baking sheet.

4 In a small bowl, mix together the salt, black pepper, oregano, and crushed red pepper.

5 Sprinkle the spice mixture evenly over the chicken pieces. Top with the provolone, prosciutto, and 2 tablespoons of parsley.

6 Roll the cutlets to enclose the filling and secure with 2 parallel skewers, placing 2 cutlets on each of the skewers.

7 Drizzle with the oil and grill for 5 minutes per side to get grill marks.

8 Transfer the skewers off direct heat and continue to grill over indirect heat for another 10 to 15 minutes, turning after 5 minutes. Temperature should register 170 degrees.

9 Remove from heat and allow to rest for 5 minutes, then remove from the skewers. Squeeze lemon over the cutlets and garnish with the remaining 1 tablespoon parsley. Serve warm.

calories	fat	protein	carbs	fiber
224	17.8g	12.3g	4.78g	1g

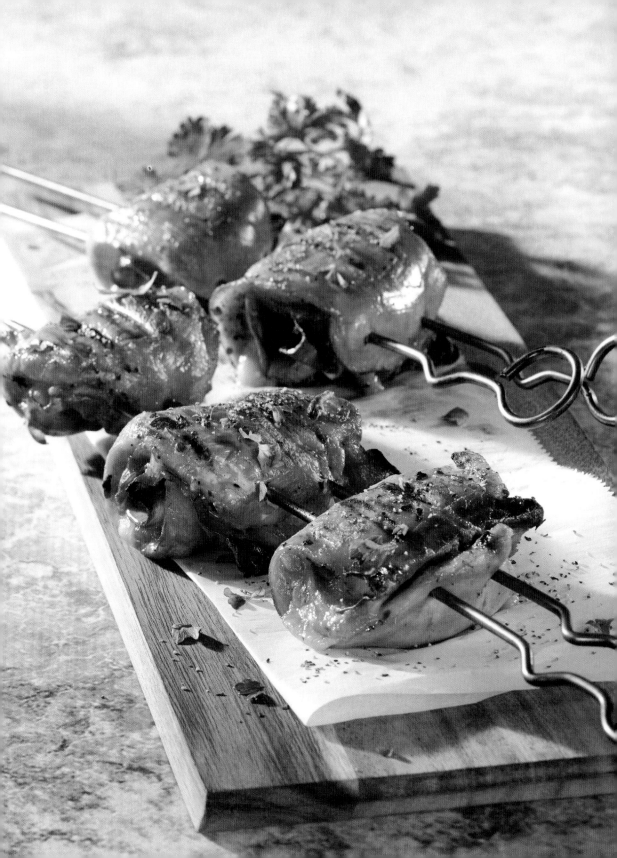

OVEN ROASTED TURKEY WITH HERBS

Yield: 12 to 14 servings

There are certain times of the year when whole turkeys are an amazing bargain. Why not spend a morning roasting one so you'll have plenty of leftovers for the freezer? It just makes delicious sense.

1 (12 to 14 pound) whole pastured turkey, thawed if frozen, with neck and giblets removed

1 teaspoon salt

1 teaspoon black pepper

8 to 10 tablespoons grass-fed butter (or ghee), softened

6 sprigs fresh rosemary

6 sprigs fresh sage

6 sprigs fresh thyme

1 Preheat the oven to 325 degrees. Lightly grease the rack of a roasting pan with olive oil cooking spray and fill the bottom of the pan with 3 cups water.

2 Place the turkey on the rack and rub all over with the salt and pepper.

3 Slip your fingers between the skin of the turkey and the meat, being careful not to rip the skin. Work the softened butter under the skin of the breast meat.

4 Place the herb sprigs in the cavity of the bird, and truss.

5 Insert a thermometer in the thigh just above the drumstick, making sure it doesn't touch the bone.

6 Place in the oven so you can easily see the thermometer through the oven window. Roast for 3½ to 4 hours or until the internal temperature reaches 160 degrees.

7 Remove from the oven and allow to rest at least 20 minutes before slicing. Cool completely before packaging for the refrigerator or freezer.

calories	fat	protein	carbs	fiber
744	41.2g	87.2g	0.81g	0.27g

SLOW COOKER RUMP ROAST

Yield: 8 to 10 servings

A slow cooker is like having an assistant in your kitchen. With just a bit of forethought, you can have a marvelous home-cooked dinner ready at the end of a long day. Since this recipe makes plenty, take advantage of the leftovers for quick lunches or soups.

1 (4 ¾ pound) boneless grass-fed beef rump roast

3 cups beef bone broth (page 38)

½ cup grass-fed butter

4 garlic cloves, peeled and minced

1 onion, peeled and chopped

2 teaspoons dried basil

2 teaspoons dried oregano

1 teaspoon garlic or onion salt

1 teaspoon black pepper

1 Place the roast in the bottom of a large (6-quart) slow cooker.

2 Add the beef broth, butter, garlic, onion, basil, oregano, salt, and pepper. Cover and cook on low for 8 hours.

3 Uncover and allow to rest 20 minutes before serving warm.

calories	fat	protein	carbs	fiber
1403	62.1g	208g	3.01g	.51g

GRILLED TO PERFECTION
FILET MIGNON STEAKS

Yield: 2 servings

When grilling choice cuts of meat, keep the "less is more" rule in mind.
That means less seasoning (only salt and pepper is needed),
less turning (only once), and no punctures with a fork (use tongs).

---

2 (6 to 8 ounces)
   filet mignon steaks

½ teaspoon salt

½ teaspoon
   black pepper

2 tablespoons
   grass-fed butter
   (or ghee), divided

1 Preheat the grill to medium-high.

2 Sprinkle the steaks on both sides evenly with the
   salt and pepper.

3 Place over direct heat and close the grill lid.
   For medium-rare, cook a total of 10 minutes;
   medium, a total of 12 minutes; and medium-well,
   a total of 14 minutes. Allow the first side to cook
   2 minutes longer than the second.

4 Remove from the grill and let rest 5 minutes.

5 Add 1 tablespoon of butter to top each fillet
   before serving.

calories	fat	protein	carbs	fiber
459	34g	37.3g	1.81g	0.29g

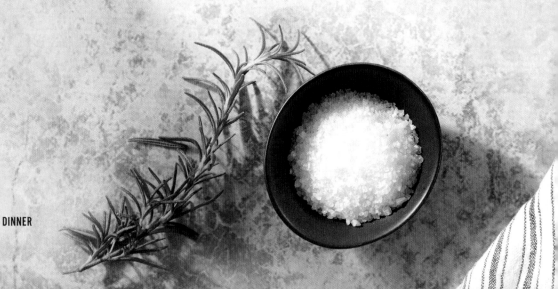

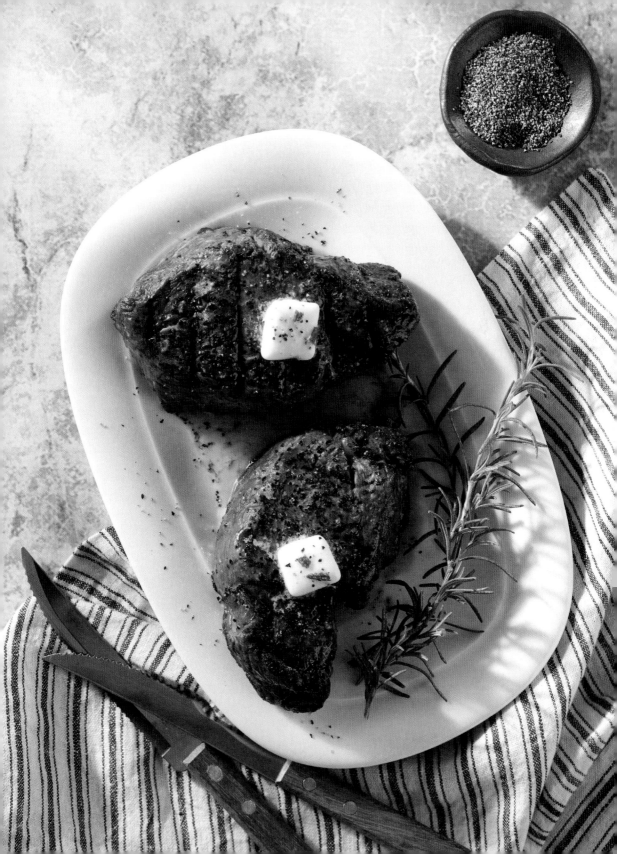

FINGER LICKING BRISKET

Yield: 8 servings

This is one of those recipes where you will want to devote a morning or afternoon to roasting. You will be rewarded with a tender, practically falling apart piece of beef that can be served anytime of day.

1 (4½ pound)
  grass-fed beef
  brisket

1 scant tablespoon salt

1 teaspoon
  white pepper

1 Preheat the oven to 350 degrees.

2 Lightly grease the rack of a roasting pan with olive oil cooking spray and add 4 cups of water to the pan.

3 Rub the brisket all over with the salt and pepper. Place it with the fat side down on the rack of the pan.

4 Cover tightly with heavy-duty aluminum foil and roast for 2 hours.

5 Discard the foil and using tongs, flip the brisket so the fat side is up.

6 Continue roasting until the brisket is fork tender and browned. This will take about 4 hours, depending on the thickness of the cut.

7 Remove pan from oven and place the brisket on a cutting board and allow it to rest at least 15 minutes. Cut across the grain on the diagonal into slices, and serve warm.

NOTE: Pair with the Tangy Barbecue Sauce (page 44).

calories	fat	protein	carbs	fiber
797	67.7g	43.3g	0.21g	0.08g

CHEESESTEAK STUFFED PEPPERS

Yield: 4 to 6 servings

*Using beautiful, large green bell peppers makes this
so lovely no one will miss the bread!*

4 large green bell peppers, halved and seeded

1 tablespoon ghee

1 pound grass-fed sirloin steak, thinly sliced

1 pound button mushrooms, wiped clean and sliced

3 medium garlic cloves, peeled and minced

3 green onions, sliced

½ teaspoon salt

¼ teaspoon black pepper

8 slices provolone cheese

1 Preheat the oven to 325 degrees.

2 Lightly coat a 13x9-inch baking dish with olive oil cooking spray.

3 Add the bell peppers with the cut side up. Bake 17 minutes.

4 Meanwhile, add the ghee to a large skillet over medium-high heat.

5 When the skillet is hot add the steak and cook 7 minutes, browning on both sides.

6 Remove the steak and place on a cutting board. Add the mushrooms to the pan. Cook 5 minutes, stirring occasionally.

7 Add the garlic, onions, salt, and pepper. Cook 2 minutes.

8 Cut the steak slices into bite-sized pieces and return to the skillet. Stir to combine and remove the skillet from heat.

9 Remove the peppers from the oven and set the broiler to high.

10 Fill the peppers with the steak mixture, pressing lightly with the back of a spoon.

11 Top each with a provolone cheese slice and broil for 3 minutes. Serve immediately.

calories	fat	protein	carbs	fiber
390	26.1g	31.7g	9.04g	2.71g

ROSEMARY CRUSTED PORK TENDERLOIN

Yield: 6 servings

Tenderloins often are sold in two-packs. Cook both for dinner and if you are lucky there will be leftovers for lunch. A plus? Your kitchen will smell marvelous!

2 (¾ to 1 pound each) pork tenderloins, trimmed

4 garlic cloves, peeled and minced

3 tablespoons avocado oil

1 tablespoon chopped fresh rosemary

1 teaspoon onion salt

½ teaspoon paprika

¼ teaspoon black pepper

1 Preheat the oven to 425 degrees.

2 Lightly grease a shallow roasting pan with olive oil cooking spray and add the tenderloins.

3 In a mixing bowl, mix together the garlic, oil, rosemary, salt, paprika, and pepper.

4 Rub the rosemary mixture all over the tops of the tenderloins. Roast 30 minutes or until an instant read thermometer registers 145 degrees.

5 Allow the pork to rest 5 minutes before slicing and serving warm.

calories	fat	protein	carbs	fiber
247	12.4g	31.4g	0.89g	0.17g

Grilled
Avocado Halves
(page 150)

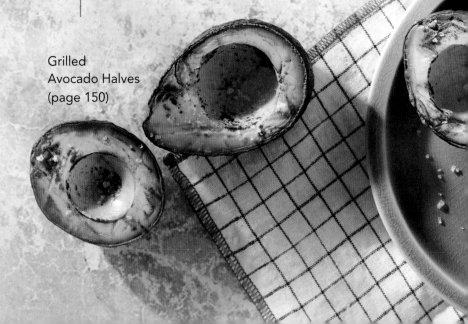

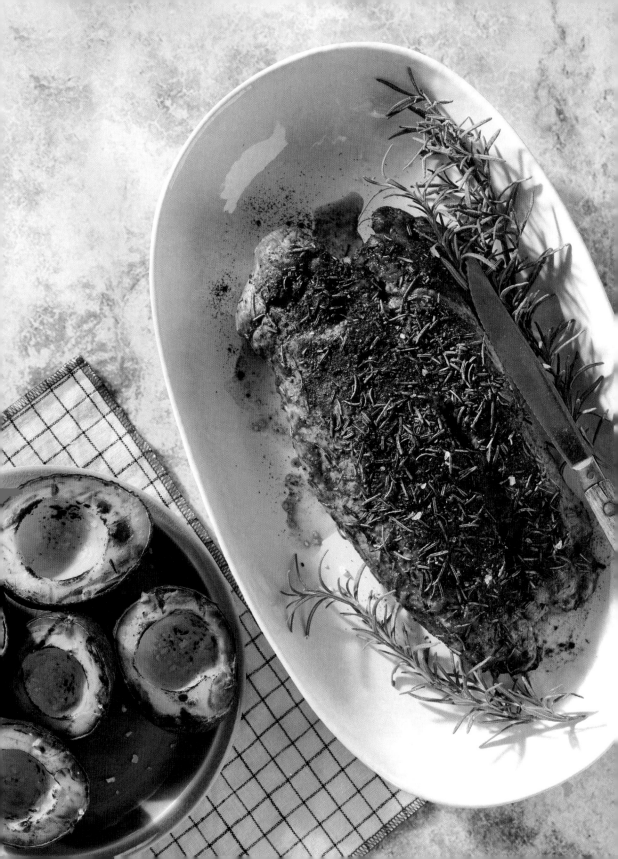

GRILLED PORK CHOPS WITH CHARRED BROCCOLI RABE

Yield: 4 servings

An aluminum foil packet of broccoli rabe cooks while the pork chops are grilled. Then the packet is carefully opened and the broccoli rabe is charred directly on the grill while the pork rests. Dinner perfection!

4 (¾-inch thick) pork loin chops

1 tablespoon lemon pepper

1¼ teaspoons onion salt, divided

1 pound broccoli rabe, trimmed

3 tablespoons olive oil

½ teaspoon garlic salt

¼ teaspoon crushed red pepper

1 Preheat the grill to medium-high.

2 Spray the pork with olive oil cooking spray on both sides. Sprinkle the pork evenly on both sides with the lemon pepper and 1 teaspoon of the onion salt. Set aside.

3 Place the broccoli rabe on a large sheet of heavy-duty aluminum foil. Drizzle with the oil and sprinkle evenly with the garlic salt, remaining ¼ teaspoon onion salt, and crushed red pepper.

4 Toss to evenly coat and fold the foil over to create a sealed packet.

5 Place the pork on the grill and after 2 minutes, rotate 45 degrees. Grill an additional 6 minutes.

6 Place the broccoli rabe packet on the grill for 8 minutes.

7 Flip the pork and grill an additional 6 minutes or until the pork is no longer pink.

8 Remove the pork and wrap in aluminum foil to rest. Remove the aluminum foil packet of broccoli rabe and carefully open away from your face to allow steam to escape.

9 Using tongs, place the broccoli rabe directly on the grill and cook 2 minutes until lightly charred. Serve warm with the pork chops.

NOTE: Serve with Hollandaise (page 42) or Tangy BBQ Sauce (page 44).

calories	fat	protein	carbs	fiber
345	17.4g	42.9g	4.4g	3.53g

FRESH HERB PORK LOIN

Yield: 8 servings

*By tying the pork loin in several places with soaked kitchen twine,
you give it a uniform shape that promotes even cooking.*

1 (4- to 4½-pound)
   pork loin, trimmed

2 teaspoons salt

1 teaspoon
   black pepper

4 garlic cloves, peeled
   and minced

4 tablespoons olive oil

1 tablespoon chopped
   fresh thyme

1 tablespoon chopped
   fresh parsley

1 tablespoon chopped
   fresh rosemary or
   oregano

1 Soak four (10-inch) pieces of kitchen twine in
   water for at least one hour before grilling.

2 Tie the pork at 3-inch intervals with the soaked
   twine. Sprinkle all over with the salt and
   pepper.

3 Using a mortar and pestle, mash together
   the garlic, oil, thyme, parsley, and rosemary
   or oregano for about 1 minute to release the
   herbs' flavors.

4 Rub the garlic mixture over the pork and set
   aside.

5 Bring one side of the grill to medium-high
   heat, around 375 degrees.

6 Place the pork on the hot side, cover, and grill
   9 minutes on each side.

7 Move the pork to the unlit side of the grill.
   Cover and grill 45 minutes or until a meat
   thermometer inserted in the center registers
   145 degrees.

8 Cover and let stand 15 minutes before slicing.
   Serve warm.

calories	fat	protein	carbs	fiber	
408	20.4g	51.8g	0.83g	0.19g	**DINNER** 143

SLOW COOKER PULLED PORK

Yield: 10 servings

Although you can use other cuts, pork shoulders make the best pulled pork. This recipe is spiced just right so you don't have to have any extra sauce. Leftovers freeze beautifully. Serve with Cauliflower and Cheese (page 148).

2 tablespoons paprika

1 tablespoon powdered stevia

1 teaspoon garlic salt

1 teaspoon black pepper

1 teaspoon onion powder

½ to 1 teaspoon cayenne, depending on taste

1 (at least 4 pounds) pork shoulder

¾ cup water

¼ cup cider vinegar

1 In a small mixing bowl, combine the paprika, stevia, salt, pepper, onion powder, and cayenne. Rub all over the pork.

2 Place the water and vinegar in the bottom of a large (6-quart) slow cooker.

3 Carefully add the pork. Cover and cook on low for 8 hours, turning once.

4 Shred the meat with 2 forks and return to slow cooker. Serve warm straight from the cooker.

NOTE: If desire, serve with Tangy BBQ Sauce (page 44).

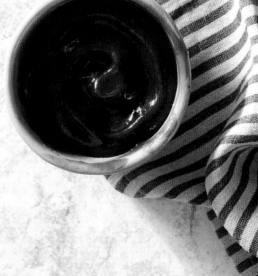

	calories	fat	protein	carbs	fiber
	436	32.8g	31.4g	2.04g	0.59g

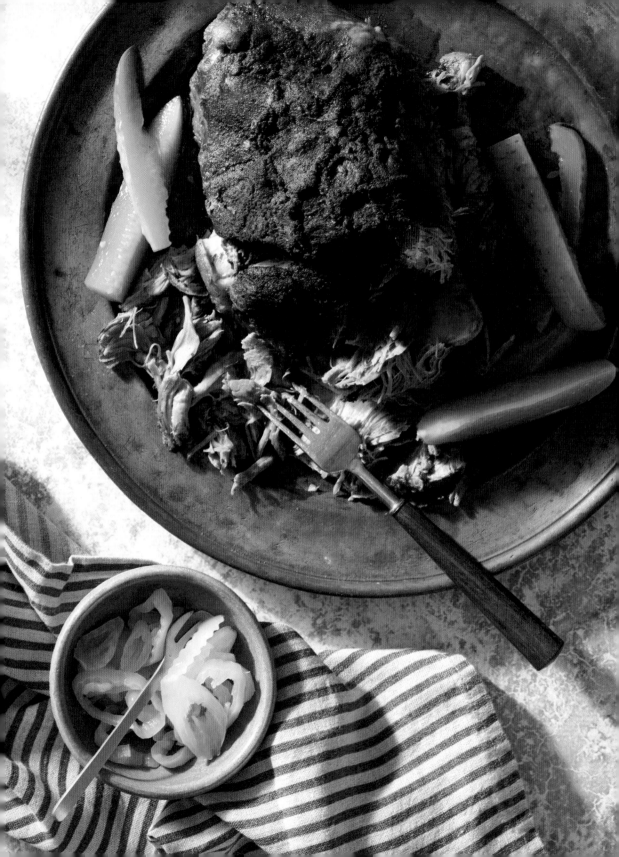

CAST IRON SKILLET HAM STEAKS

Yield: 4 servings

*If you only had room for one skillet in your kitchen, select cast iron.
It conducts heat perfectly and lasts more than a lifetime.
Pay close attention to the thickness of the ham steak called for in this recipe.
You don't want to purchase one that is too thin.*

1 (2- to 2½ pound)
ham steak,
one inch thick

2 tablespoons
grass-fed butter
(or ghee), divided

1 Place 1 tablespoon butter in a large, cast iron skillet over medium-high heat. Carefully tilt the skillet to evenly coat the bottom.

2 Add the ham steak and cook 3 minutes.

3 Remove the ham from the skillet and add the remaining 1 tablespoon butter to the skillet.

4 When the butter is melted, return the ham to the skillet, flipping to cook the other side. Cook 3 minutes and serve warm.

calories	fat	protein	carbs	fiber
362	16.6g	50g	0g	0g

BACON & BRUSSELS SPROUTS CARBONARA

Yield: 4 servings

Traditionally a spaghetti dish, this one uses shredded brussels sprouts instead. If desired, substitute pancetta for the bacon.

8 slices nitrate-free bacon

1 pound brussels sprouts, shredded

2 large garlic cloves, peeled and minced

¼ teaspoon crushed red pepper

2 eggs

½ cup grated Romano or Parmesan cheese

½ teaspoon salt

¼ teaspoon black pepper

1 Place the bacon in a large skillet over medium heat and brown on both sides, working in batches. With tongs, move the bacon to a paper towel-lined plate and allow to cool. Reserve the grease in the pan.

2 Once the bacon has cooled, crumble the bacon to pieces.

3 Add the brussels sprouts, garlic, and crushed red pepper to the skillet with the reserved bacon grease. Cook, stirring frequently, for 8 to 9 minutes.

4 Meanwhile, in a small bowl whisk together the eggs, Romano or Parmesan cheese, salt, and pepper. Stir in the crumbled bacon.

5 Remove the skillet from the heat and slowly add the egg mixture, stirring continuously for 2 minutes or until the egg sauce thickens. Serve immediately.

calories	fat	protein	carbs	fiber
275	18.2g	21.6g	6.19g	1.77g

MOZZARELLA PIZZA CRUST

Yield: 6 to 8 slices

This crust will reheat very well if you get ambitious and want to make extra.

2 cups shredded mozzarella cheese

¾ cup almond flour

2 tablespoons garlic and herb cream cheese, at room temperature

1 egg, at room temperature and beaten

1 teaspoon Italian seasoning

¼ teaspoon onion salt

¼ teaspoon white pepper

1   Preheat the oven to 350 degrees. Place a large piece of parchment paper on a flat surface and set another piece of parchment paper aside.

2   In a microwavable bowl, combine the mozzarella cheese and flour, stirring well to coat the cheese.

3   Make a well in the center of the flour mixture and add the cream cheese. Microwave for 1 minute, stir, then microwave for another 30 seconds.

4   Stir in the egg, Italian seasoning, salt, and pepper, blending well to form a dough.

5   Transfer the dough onto one sheet of the parchment paper. It will look and feel wet.

6   Place the second piece of parchment paper on top and with a rolling pin, roll to between ¼ and ½ inch thickness.

7   Remove and discard the top piece of parchment paper and, leaving the dough on the bottom parchment paper, transfer to a pizza stone. With a fork, poke several holes in the top of the crust.

8   Bake 13 to 15 minutes or until the crust is starting to brown.

9   Remove from the oven and add the toppings of your choice, if desired, or slice and enjoy plain.

10 If toppings are added, bake an additional 5 minutes or until bubbly.

11 Allow to rest 2 minutes before slicing and serving warm.

NOTE: Enjoy topped with keto-friendly favorites such as green peppers, tomatoes, artichoke hearts, mushrooms, cheese, or pesto.

calories	fat	protein	carbs	fiber
166	13.4g	9.5g	3.23g	1.19g

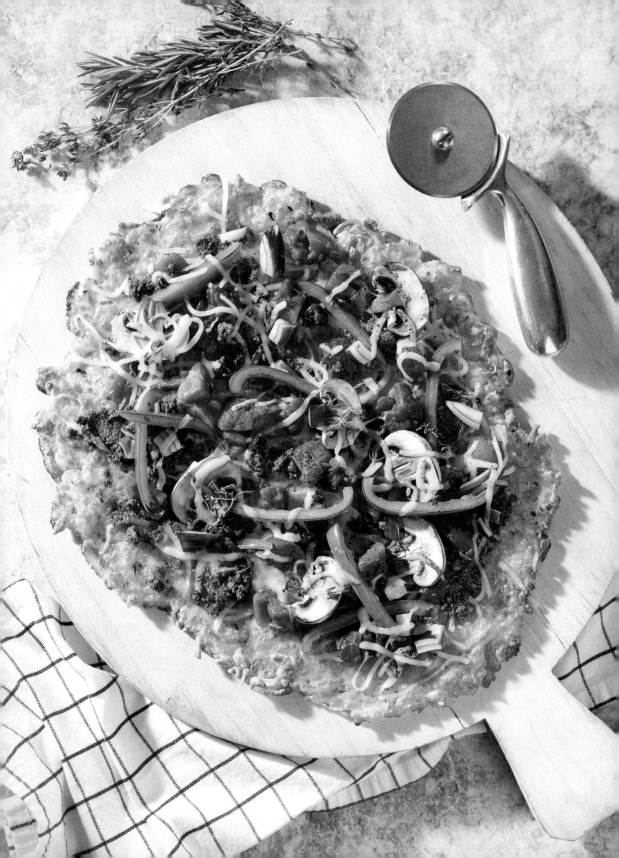

CAULIFLOWER AND CHEESE

Yield: 6 to 8 servings

*You won't even miss the "m" word when you take a bite
of this heavenly side dish. Turn it into a complete meal
by adding cooked ham before spreading over the cauliflower.*

1 large head
cauliflower, trimmed
and cut into florets

3 ounces
cream cheese

½ cup sour cream

¼ cup grated
Parmesan cheese

2 tablespoons
heavy cream

2 garlic cloves, peeled
and minced

2 green onions,
chopped

½ teaspoon onion salt

¼ teaspoon
black pepper

⅛ teaspoon cayenne

1 cup grated sharp
Cheddar cheese

1 Preheat the oven to 350 degrees.

2 Meanwhile, place the cauliflower in a large
pot of boiling water and cook for 5 minutes.
Drain and place in a 9x13-inch baking dish
lightly greased with olive oil cooking spray.

3 In a medium mixing bowl, combine the cream
cheese, sour cream, Parmesan cheese, cream,
garlic, onions, salt, pepper, and cayenne. Blend
well and spread evenly over the cauliflower.

4 Top with the Cheddar cheese and bake
uncovered for 20 minutes. Let rest 5 minutes
before serving warm.

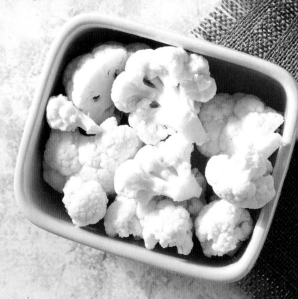

calories	fat	protein	carbs	fiber
195	15.5g	8.23g	7.54g	2.45g

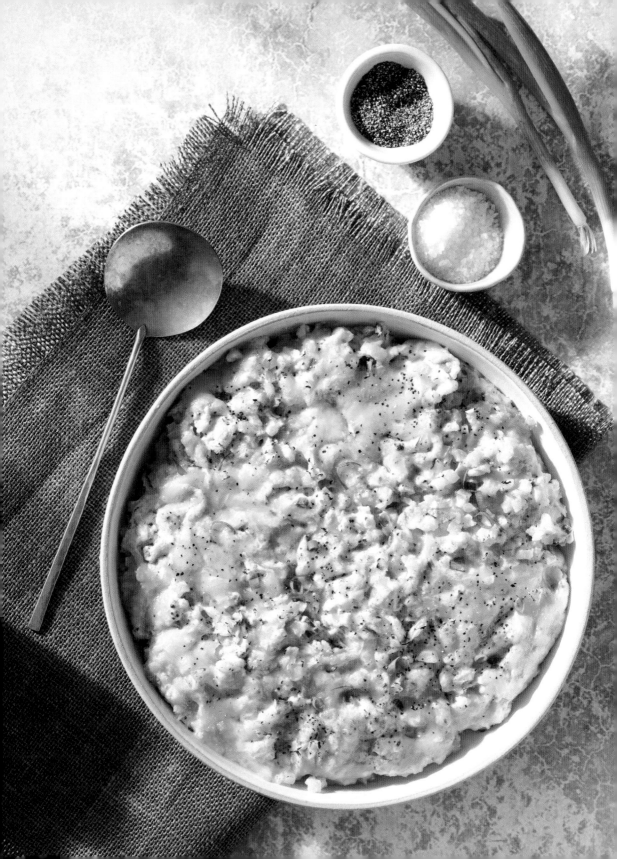

GRILLED AVOCADO HALVES

Yield: 4 servings

Serve this creamy deliciousness as a side dish or as a topping over microgreens. Just throw them on the grill when cooking meat and in less than 5 minutes, lunch is on!

2 ripe avocados,
   pitted and halved

2 tablespoons
   lime juice, divided

1 tablespoon
   avocado or olive oil

½ teaspoon
   garlic salt

1 Preheat the grill to medium-high.

2 Brush the avocados' cut edges with
   1 tablespoon lime juice, then brush with oil.

3 Gently place the cut sides down, and grill for
   3 minutes.

4 Remove and immediately sprinkle with the salt.
   Let stand 5 minutes. Brush with the remaining
   1 tablespoon lime juice before serving.

NOTE: Add a spoonful of Salsa Verde (page 51) or
Roasted Salsa (page 182) to heighten flavors.

calories	fat	protein	carbs	fiber
194	18.2g	2.04g	9.22g	6.76g

EASY CAPRESE SALAD

Yield: 2 servings

*This recipe can be ready in under 10 minutes and is a beautiful
side dish to complement most chicken or fish dishes.
Or add some leafy green lettuce and you have a lovely lunchtime salad.*

½ pound grape tomatoes, halved

½ pound fresh mozzarella, cubed (or can buy container of bocconcini)

6 large fresh basil leaves, chopped

4 tablespoons olive oil

2 teaspoons balsamic vinegar

¼ teaspoon salt

Black pepper to taste

1   In a small bowl, toss tomatoes, mozzarella, chopped basil, salt, and oil together.

2   Drizzle with balsamic vinegar and a dash of pepper to taste. Serve as a side dish or over lettuce as a salad.

calories	fat	protein	carbs	fiber
604	52.6g	26.2g	7.84g	1.39g

CREAMED SPINACH

Yield: 4 servings

*This is a filling side dish that pairs well with grilled seafood.
Or use it as a dip!*

4 tablespoons avocado oil, divided

1 large shallot, peeled and chopped

1 large garlic clove, peeled and minced

¼ cup chicken bone broth (page 38)

1 pound fresh baby spinach, coarsely chopped

3 ounces cream cheese, cubed and softened

⅛ teaspoon garlic salt

⅛ teaspoon black pepper

⅛ teaspoon cayenne

1 Place 2 tablespoons of oil in a large skillet over medium-high heat.

2 Add the shallot and garlic and sauté 5 minutes, stirring occasionally.

3 Add the broth and remaining 2 tablespoons of oil. When it begins to simmer, add the spinach, one handful at a time. Cook 4 minutes and add the cream cheese, salt, pepper, and cayenne.

4 Stir constantly until the cream cheese melts completely. Serve warm.

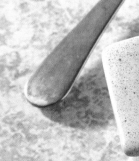

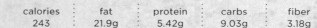

calories	fat	protein	carbs	fiber
243	21.9g	5.42g	9.03g	3.18g

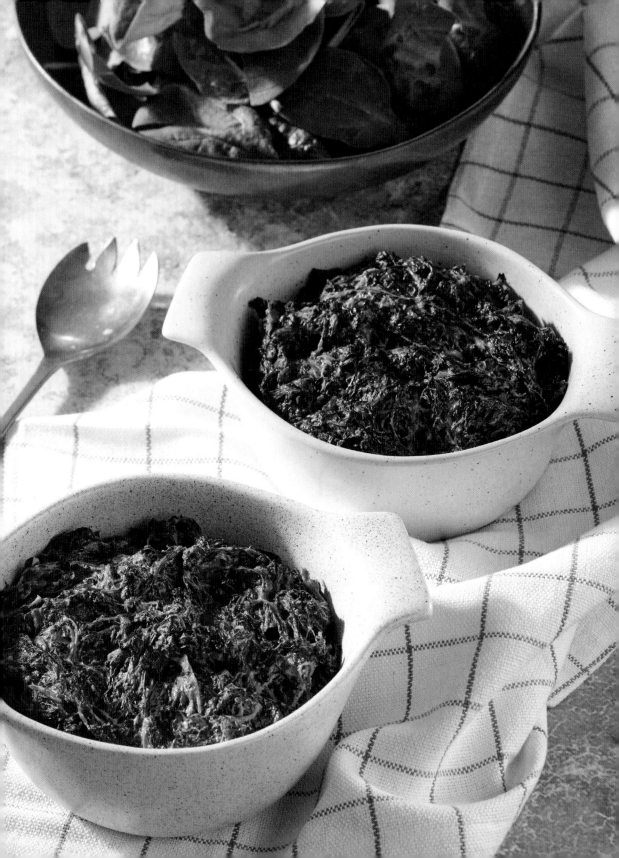

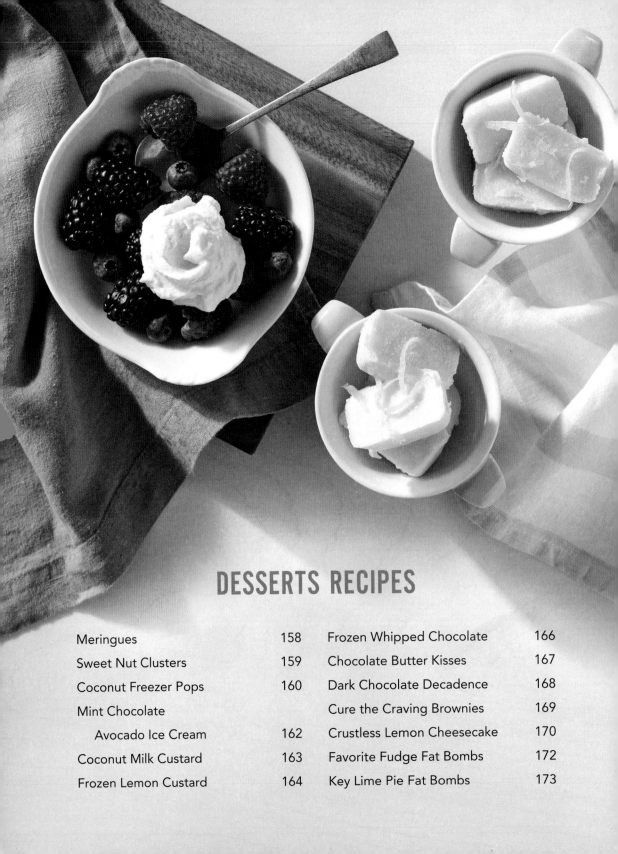

DESSERTS RECIPES

DESSERTS

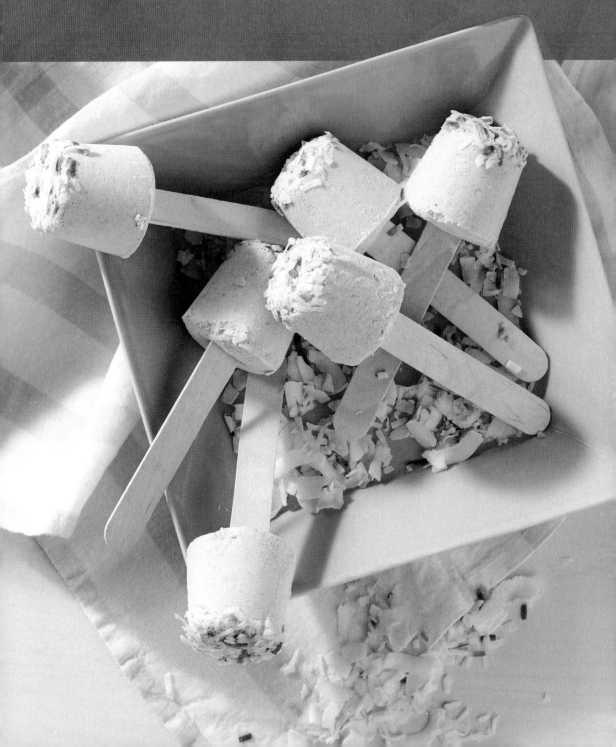

MERINGUES

Yield: 22 meringues

*Powdered erythritol is available at most supermarkets
and is a natural sugar substitute.
It is available in both granular and powdered forms.*

2 egg whites

¼ teaspoon
  cream of tartar

½ teaspoon pure
  almond extract

¼ cup powdered
  erythritol

1 Preheat the oven to 200 degrees. Line a baking sheet with parchment paper and set aside.

2 In the bowl of an electric mixer, beat the egg whites on medium speed until frothy.

3 Add the cream of tartar and almond extract, and increase the mixer speed to high.

4 After soft peaks have formed, gradually and slowly add the powdered erythritol, 1 tablespoon at a time, to the egg mixture. Continue beating until stiff peaks have formed.

5 With a spoon or piping bag, place dollops of the mixture on the prepared pan, about the size of a tablespoon.

6 Bake for 1 hour, then turn off the oven and leave in the oven for 1 ½ hours longer. Do not open the oven door.

7 Remove and serve, or transfer to an airtight container.

VARIATIONS: Substitute an equal amount of lemon, vanilla, peppermint, orange, banana, mint, black walnut, raspberry, coconut, or coffee extract for the almond extract if desired.

Serving size: 2 pieces

calories	fat	protein	carbs	fiber
3.06	0.01g	0.65g	0.09g	0g

SWEET NUT CLUSTERS

Yield: 6 to 8 servings

Cardamom has a spicy citrus flavor and is perfect for adding flavor and aroma. Use any nuts you desire to make this sweet treat.

1 egg white

1 teaspoon liquid stevia

1 teaspoon ground cinnamon

1 teaspoon ground ginger

¼ teaspoon ground cardamom

1 cup raw whole almonds

1 cup raw pumpkin seeds

1 Preheat the oven to 350 degrees and line a baking sheet with parchment paper. Set aside.

2 In a small mixing bowl, whisk together the egg white, stevia, cinnamon, ginger, and cardamom for 1 minute.

3 Stir in the almonds and pumpkin seeds, tossing to evenly coat.

4 Spread on the prepared pan and bake for 20 minutes.

5 Place on a wire rack to cool completely, around 30 minutes.

6 Break into bite-sized pieces, and store in an airtight container.

calories	fat	protein	carbs	fiber
299	25.5g	12.7g	10.3g	5.01g

COCONUT FREEZER POPS

Yield: 6 to 8 freezer pops

You can quickly and easily change the flavor of these treats to fit your mood. Simply change the extract flavors. You can also substitute pecan butter for the almond butter.

¼ cup coconut butter

¼ cup almond butter

½ teaspoon liquid stevia

½ teaspoon pure coconut extract

Pinch of salt

1 cup unsweetened full-fat Greek yogurt

6 to 8 3-ounce paper cups

wooden craft sticks

1. In the bowl of an electric mixer, blend together the coconut butter, almond butter, stevia, coconut extract, and salt. Reduce the mixer speed to low and add the yogurt.

2. Spoon the mixture into the paper cups, filling two-thirds full.

3. Place in the freezer for 1 hour and add the wooden craft sticks in the center.

4. Continue to freeze for 4 hours or until solid.

5. To serve, peel off the paper cup and serve immediately.

calories	fat	protein	carbs	fiber
144	11.7g	5.36g	5.04g	2.08g

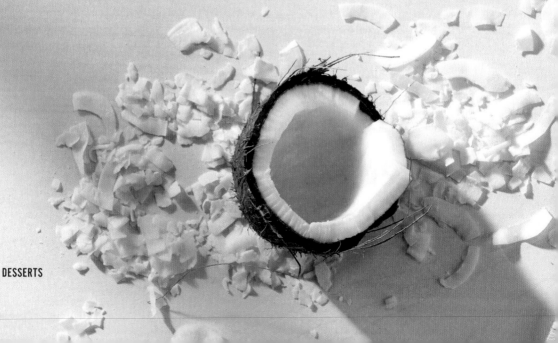

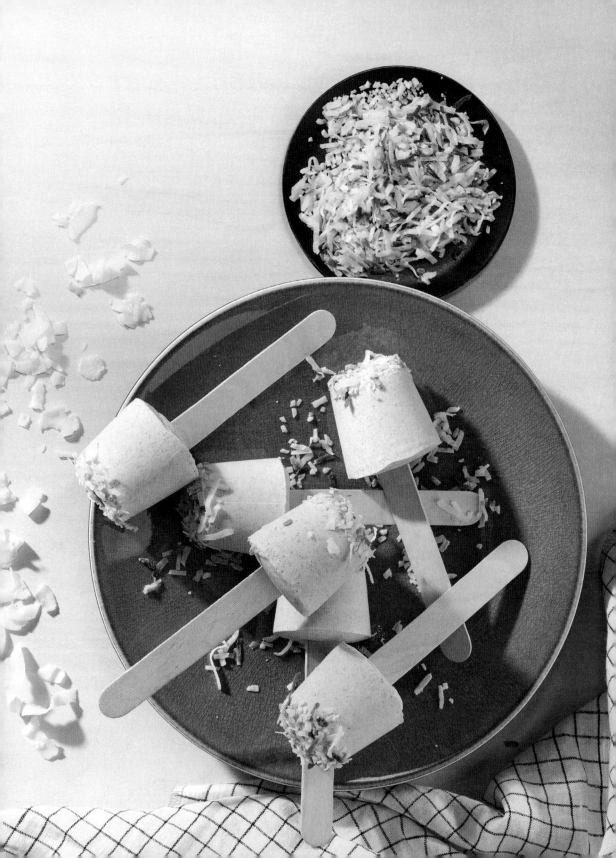

MINT CHOCOLATE
AVOCADO ICE CREAM

Yield: 6 servings

This recipe just seems wrong when you see its name, but the velvety consistency of avocados makes this frozen dessert taste rich and creamy. It can easily be doubled if serving a crowd.

3 ripe avocados, pitted and peeled

Coconut Cream from 1 (14.5-ounce) can (page 40)

¼ cup powdered stevia

6 tablespoons coconut oil

½ teaspoon pure mint extract*

¼ cup cacao nibs

1 In a blender, purée the avocados, Coconut Cream, stevia, oil, and mint extract* until smooth.

2 Stir in the cacao nibs and transfer to an electric ice cream freezer.

3 Follow the manufacturer's directions for freezing.

*VARIATIONS: Replace the mint extract with vanilla, almond, coconut, banana, or flavor of your choice.

calories	fat	protein	carbs	fiber
437	42.9g	4.02g	17.6g	7.01g

COCONUT MILK CUSTARD

Yield: 2 servings

*This individually served dessert is just right for a special occasion.
It can be consumed at room temperature or chilled.*

¾ cup canned
   coconut milk

2 egg yolks

2 tablespoons
   coconut oil

1 teaspoon
   liquid stevia

¼ teaspoon
   pure vanilla extract

¼ teaspoon pure
   coconut extract

1 tablespoon
   sliced almonds

1 Preheat the oven to 300 degrees. Lightly grease 2 ramekins with olive oil cooking spray and set aside.

2 Place the coconut milk in a small saucepan over medium heat and bring to a simmer.

3 Meanwhile, whisk the egg yolks in a small bowl.

4 When the milk is steaming (not bubbling), pour approximately ⅛ cup of the hot milk slowly into the egg yolks whisking constantly. Slowly add the rest of the hot coconut milk to the egg yolks gradually bringing the egg yolk mixture up in temperature.

5 Add the stevia, vanilla, and coconut extracts.

6 Evenly divide mixture between the prepared ramekins and bake 25 to 30 minutes or until just set.

7 Remove from the oven and place on a wire rack to cool slightly.

8 Place the almonds on an ungreased baking sheet and toast in the oven as it cools.

9 After 15 minutes, sprinkle the almonds on top of the custards and serve.

calories	fat	protein	carbs	fiber
248	23.5g	4.35g	6.16g	0.87g

FROZEN LEMON CUSTARD

Yield: 3 to 4 servings

This dessert is a rich tasting, lemony sherbet type treat.
For a key lime twist, substitute lime juice for the lemon juice.
If desired, freeze in an ice cube tray for easy, quick treats..

4 eggs

½ cup grass-fed butter

½ cup lemon juice

2 teaspoons powdered
stevia

2 teaspoons
unflavored
powdered gelatin

1 Place the eggs, butter, lemon juice, stevia, and gelatin in a medium saucepan over low heat.

2 Stir frequently. When the mixture comes to a simmer, remove from heat.

3 Set aside to cool for 20 minutes.

4 Transfer to a shallow container and freeze for at least 3 hours.

calories	fat	protein	carbs	fiber
250	23.5g	4.33g	7.81g	0.79g

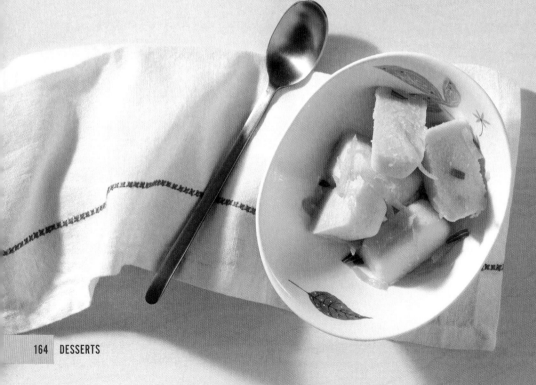

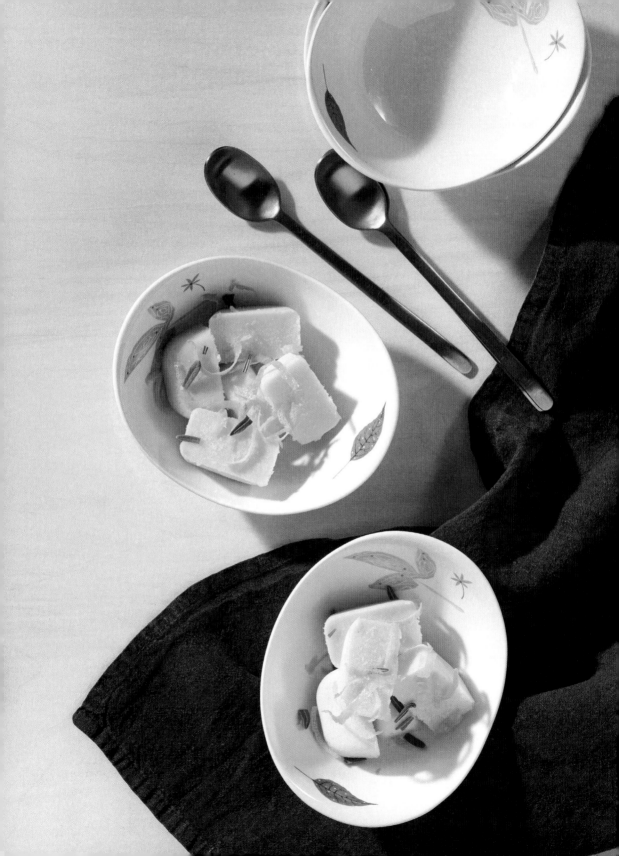

FROZEN WHIPPED CHOCOLATE

Yield: 2 servings

Although you can serve this simply chilled, it's best frozen.

½ cup heavy whipping cream

1 tablespoon unsweetened cocoa

1 tablespoon almond butter

1 tablespoon MCT oil powder

1 teaspoon powdered stevia

1 Place the cream, cocoa, butter, MCT oil powder, and stevia in a blender. Whip at high speed until smooth.

2 Transfer to a shallow container, cover, and freeze for at least 3 hours.

calories	fat	protein	carbs	fiber
294	29.8g	3.9g	6.14g	3.32g

CHOCOLATE BUTTER KISSES

Yield: 20 pieces

This is a really easy dessert that only needs refrigeration.
Try to keep the dollops no larger than 1-inch in diameter.

½ cup
coconut butter

½ cup
grass-fed butter,
softened

¼ cup coconut oil

3 tablespoons
unsweetened cocoa

1 teaspoon powdered
stevia

1 Place the coconut butter, butter, oil, cocoa,
and stevia in a food processor and process
until smooth.

2 Line a baking sheet with parchment paper and
spoon 1-inch dollops onto the sheet.

3 Refrigerate until solid, then serve or transfer to
a shallow covered container and store in the
refrigerator.

Serving size: 1 piece

calories	fat	protein	carbs	fiber
107	11g	0.61g	1.82g	1.1g

DARK CHOCOLATE DECADENCE

Yield: 6 servings

The name says it all!

2 cups heavy whipping cream, divided

1 tablespoon powdered gelatin

1 cup almond milk, at room temperature

½ cup powdered erythritol

½ cup unsweetened cocoa

1 teaspoon pure vanilla extract

1 Place ¼ cup of the cream in the mixing bowl of a stand mixer and sprinkle the gelatin over the top. Set aside.

2 Place the remaining 1 ¾ cream and almond milk in a heavy saucepan over medium heat. Allow to reach a slight simmer, around 4 minutes.

3 Meanwhile, add the powdered erythritol and cocoa to the gelatin mixture, and whisk until well blended.

4 Place on the stand mixer on low speed. Gradually add the warm milk mixture until combined.

5 Increase the mixer speed to medium-low and add the vanilla extract.

6 Pour into 6 ramekins and refrigerate 1 hour.

7 After 1 hour, cover the tops with plastic wrap and refrigerate 1 hour more. Serve or transfer to freezer.

NOTE: Can also be frozen for up to one month.

calories	fat	protein	carbs	fiber
188	15.9g	3.35g	12g	2.65g

CURE THE CRAVING BROWNIES

Yield: 9 brownies

You don't need to throw in the towel when it comes to desserts when on the Keto Zone diet. This brownie recipe is sure to satisfy your sweet tooth in the best way. The key to getting these brownies just right is to mix at a low speed and let the batter rest.

1 cup almond or coconut butter

3 large eggs, room temperature

½ cup cocoa powder

¾ cup powdered erythritol

1½ tablespoons coconut flour

Pinch of sea salt

2 tablespoons 85% dark chocolate chunks (optional)

2 tablespoons chopped almonds, walnuts, or pecans. (optional)

1 Preheat the oven to 325 degrees. Line a 9x9 inch baking dish with parchment paper and lightly grease with olive oil cooking spray.

2 In the bowl of a stand mixer, add the almond butter and eggs. Blend at a low speed until smooth.

3 Add the cocoa powder, erythritol, coconut flour, and sea salt. Blend at a low speed until combined.

4 If adding, fold in chocolate chunks or nuts. Do not overmix.

5 Let the batter sit for 4 minutes.

6 Transfer the batter to the lined baking dish and smooth with a spatula. Bake for 15 minutes and check. Brownies should no longer be wet, but shouldn't look dry. Bake in additional 2 minute increments as needed.

7 Remove from oven and let cool completely before cutting and serving. Cover leftovers with plastic wrap and store on the counter.

calories	fat	protein	carbs	fiber
231	19.2g	9.32g	10.4g	5.53g

CRUSTLESS LEMON CHEESECAKE

Yield: 10 servings

This cheesecake has all the creamy texture and lemon flavor you crave without the carb-loaded crust. You won't miss it!

3 (8-ounce) packages cream cheese, softened

1 cup sour cream

⅓ cup Swerve

3 eggs

1 egg yolk

1 teaspoon pure lemon extract

1 teaspoon lemon juice

1 teaspoon liquid stevia

1 teaspoon baking powder

¼ teaspoon salt

1 Preheat the oven to 325 degrees. Grease the bottom of an 8-inch springform pan with olive oil cooking spray and wrap the outside of the pan with aluminum foil. Set aside.

2 In the bowl of an electric mixer, combine the cream cheese, sour cream, Swerve, eggs, egg yolk, lemon extract, lemon juice, stevia, baking powder, and salt. Beat for 2 minutes.

3 Transfer the mixture to the prepared springform pan. Place in a separate, larger roasting pan and fill with hot water halfway up the sides of the cheesecake pan being careful to keep the water level below the aluminum foil.

4 Bake for 45 minutes and turn off the oven. Allow the cheesecake to sit in the oven for 1 hour without opening the door or disturbing the pan.

5 Remove the cheesecake from the oven and the water bath. Remove the aluminum foil.

6 Refrigerate at least 4 hours. Remove from springform pan before slicing and serving.

NOTE: Top with ¼ of berries of choice (blackberries, raspberries, blueberries, or strawberries), lemon slices or zest of a lemon, or a dollop of Coconut Whipped Cream (page 40).

calories	fat	protein	carbs	fiber
324	29.8g	6.9g	8.7g	0.02g

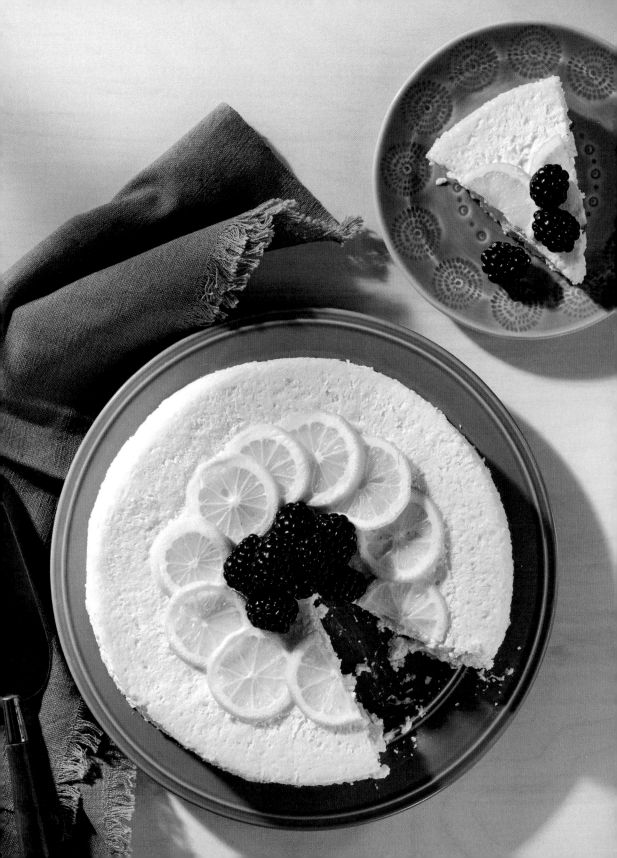

FAVORITE FUDGE FAT BOMBS

Yields: 30 fat bombs, approximately

Fat bombs are an excellent source of adding fat to your day to keep you in the Keto Zone. This fudge fat bomb recipe is very versatile, so try it with different nut butters or dark chocolate chunks.

1 cup almond butter

¾ cup coconut oil

1 tablespoon
    MCT oil powder

½ cup unsweetened
    cocoa powder

⅓ cup coconut flour

½ teaspoon
    liquid stevia

Pinch of sea salt

1 Heat a saucepan over medium heat and combine the almond butter and coconut oil.

2 Once melted, remove from heat and add the MCT powder, cocoa powder, coconut flour, stevia, and pinch of salt to the pan. Stir until well combined.

3 Allow mixture to cool slightly and taste. Add additional stevia if needed, starting with one or two drops.

4 Lightly grease 2 ice cube trays with olive oil cooking spray.

5 Pour mixture into 2 ice cube trays, filling each compartment about halfway, and transfer to the freezer. Freeze for 2–3 hours.

6 Store in the freezer and serve cold.

Serving size: 1 bomb

calories	fat	protein	carbs	fiber
111	10.6g	2.2g	3.15g	1.94g

KEY LIME PIE FAT BOMBS

Yields: 30 fat bombs, approximately

Key lime pie, meet fat bomb. Fat bomb, meet key lime pie.
This twist on a classic recipe is still tart and creamy, just as a key lime pie
should be. When you're craving something sweet and tangy,
look no further than this Keto treat!

½ cup
macadamia nuts

¼ cup sunflower
seeds, shelled

⅓ cup coconut oil,
melted

½ teaspoon
liquid stevia

¼ cup unsweetened
coconut milk

3 tablespoons
lime juice

1 tablespoon
coconut flour

1 teaspoon lime zest

1 Add the macadamia nuts, sunflower seeds,
coconut oil, stevia, coconut milk, lime juice,
and coconut flower in the bowl of a food
processor.

2 Pulse until well-blended and mixture is thick
and creamy.

3 Taste test and add additional stevia, if needed,
starting with one or two drops.

4 Fold lime zest into mixture.

5 Lightly grease 2 ice cube trays with olive oil
cooking spray.

6 Divide mixture into ice tube trays, filling
each compartment about halfway.
Freeze for 1 to 2 hours.

7 Store in the freezer and serve cold.

Serving size: 1 bomb

calories	fat	protein	carbs	fiber
45	4.8g	0.34g	0.8g	0.36g

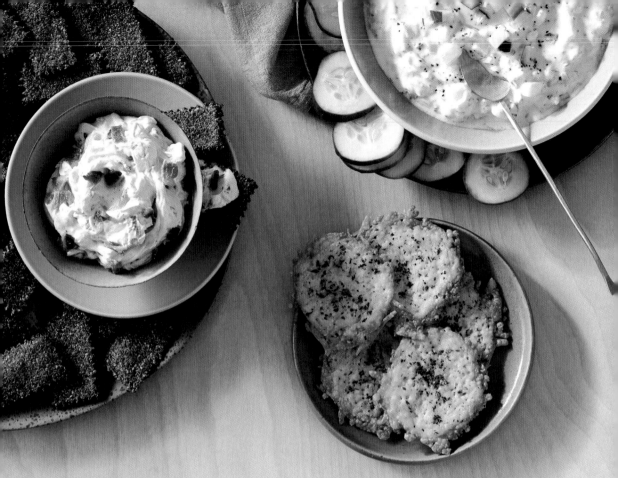

SNACKS RECIPES

SNACKS

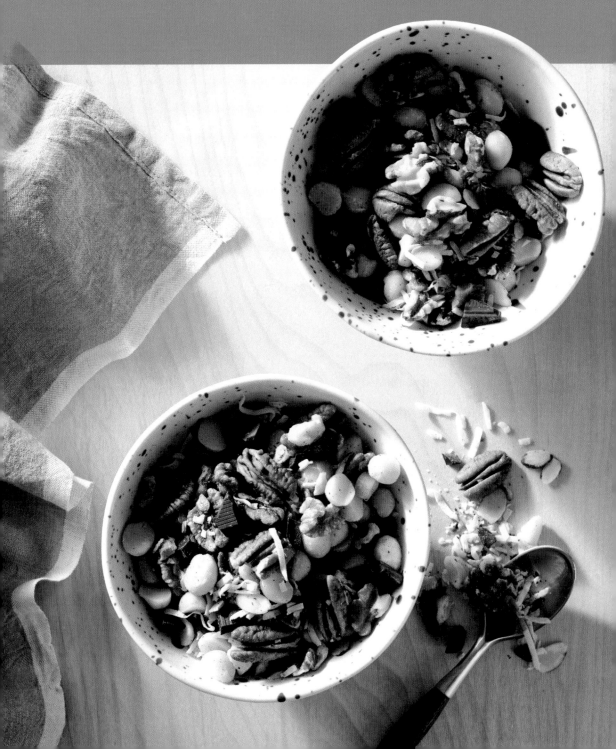

ADDICTIVE GUACAMOLE

Yield: 6 servings

This recipe is so easy you can make and serve it immediately.
If you need to prepare it ahead of time, make sure you place plastic wrap
directly on the surface of the guacamole and refrigerate until ready to serve.

3 avocados, pitted
and peeled

1 large shallot, peeled
and chopped

2 large garlic cloves,
peeled and minced

¼ cup chopped
cilantro

1 tablespoon
lime juice

1 tablespoon
avocado oil

1 tablespoon
crushed red pepper

1 teaspoon salt

¼ teaspoon
white pepper

1 In a medium bowl, mash the avocados with a
fork to the desired consistency.

2 Stir in the shallot, garlic, cilantro, lime juice, oil,
crushed red pepper, salt, and pepper.

3 Blend well and serve immediately.

calories	fat	protein	carbs	fiber
196	17.2g	2.5g	12g	7.5g

SPINACH ARTICHOKE DIP

Yield: 6 to 8 servings

*This recipe has slowly become a classic, but this version has no guilt!
It is delicious warm but can also be served straight from
the refrigerator or at room temperature.*

1 (8-ounce) package plain or chive
cream cheese, softened

1 cup sour cream

½ cup grated Romano or Parmesan
cheese, divided

3 garlic cloves, peeled and minced

1 small onion, peeled and chopped

¼ teaspoon onion or garlic salt

¼ teaspoon black pepper

⅛ teaspoon paprika

⅛ teaspoon cayenne

1 (10-ounce) package frozen, chopped
spinach, thawed and squeezed dry

1 (9-ounce) package frozen artichoke
hearts, thawed, squeezed dry, and
chopped

1 Preheat the oven to 350 degrees.

2 Lightly grease an 8-inch square baking dish with olive oil cooking spray
and set aside.

3 In the bowl of an electric mixer, combine the cream cheese, sour cream,
¼ cup Romano or Parmesan cheese, garlic, onion, salt, pepper, paprika,
and cayenne on medium speed until smooth.

4 Stir in the spinach and artichoke hearts until well blended.

5 Transfer to the prepared baking dish. Top with the remaining ¼ cup cheese.

6 Bake 18 to 20 minutes or until bubbly.

7 Let stand 5 minutes before serving warm.

calories	fat	protein	carbs	fiber
258	22g	8.5g	9.1g	2.6g

APPLEWOOD BACON DIP

Yield: ⅔ cup

*Spread this delicious dip on celery sticks or on
Garlic Flaxseed Crackers (page 184).*

4 slices nitrate-free
applewood smoked
bacon

4 ounces jalapeño
cream cheese,
softened

2 tablespoons
heavy whipping
cream

1 teaspoon chopped
fresh chives

¼ teaspoon
black pepper

Fresh parsley,
chopped for garnish

1 Place the bacon in a large skillet over
medium-high heat.

2 Cook until crisp and drain on paper towels.
Remove skillet from heat and reserve the bacon
grease in the skillet. Crumble when the bacon
is cool enough to handle.

3 Meanwhile, in a medium mixing bowl, combine
the cream cheese, cream, chives, and pepper.

4 Add 1 teaspoon of the reserved bacon grease
and blend well.

5 Stir in the bacon and top with fresh the parsley.

6 Serve immediately or refrigerate for later use.

Serving size: ⅓ cup

calories	fat	protein	carbs	fiber
280	23.5g	12.3g	7g	0.1g

CREAMY SEAFOOD DIP

Yield: 6 servings

*Tiny salad shrimp and lump crab meat combine to give
this dip personality. Serve it warm or cool to room temperature.
For an extra kick, use jalapeño cream cheese.*

1 (8-ounce) package
cream cheese,
softened

1 small green bell
pepper, seeded and
chopped

2 garlic cloves, peeled
and minced

2 tablespoon
avocado mayonnaise

1 tablespoon
horseradish

½ teaspoon
black pepper

¼ teaspoon
onion salt

¼ teaspoon cayenne

½ pound
lump crab meat

½ pound small salad
shrimp

1 Preheat the oven to 350 degrees.

2 Lightly grease a 9-inch pie pan with olive oil
cooking spray and set aside.

3 In a mixing bowl, blend together the cream
cheese, bell pepper, garlic, mayonnaise,
horseradish, pepper, salt, and cayenne.

4 Gently fold in the crab meat and shrimp.

5 Transfer to the prepared baking dish and
spread evenly.

6 Bake 20 minutes or until bubbly. Serve warm.

calories	fat	protein	carbs	fiber
257	19.4g	16.5g	4.07g	0.46g

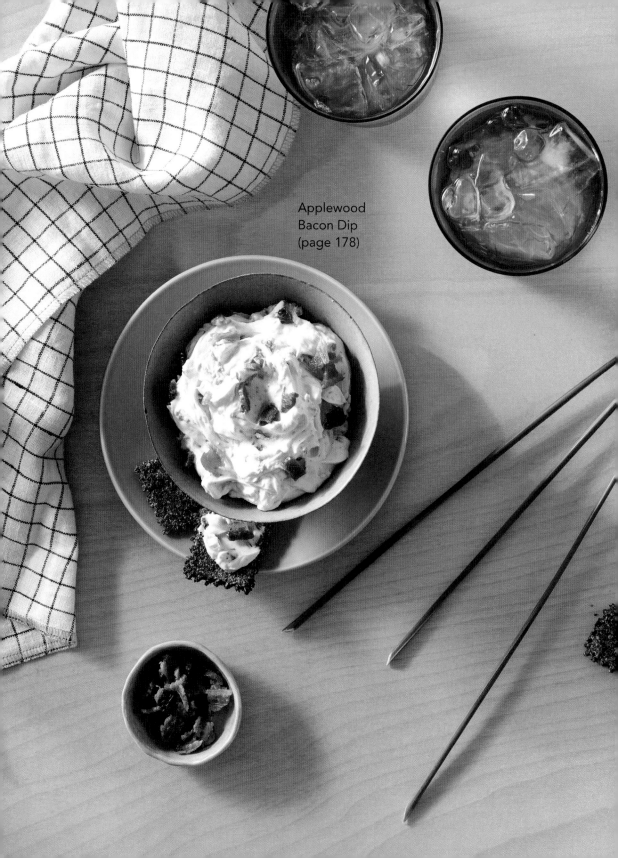

Applewood
Bacon Dip
(page 178)

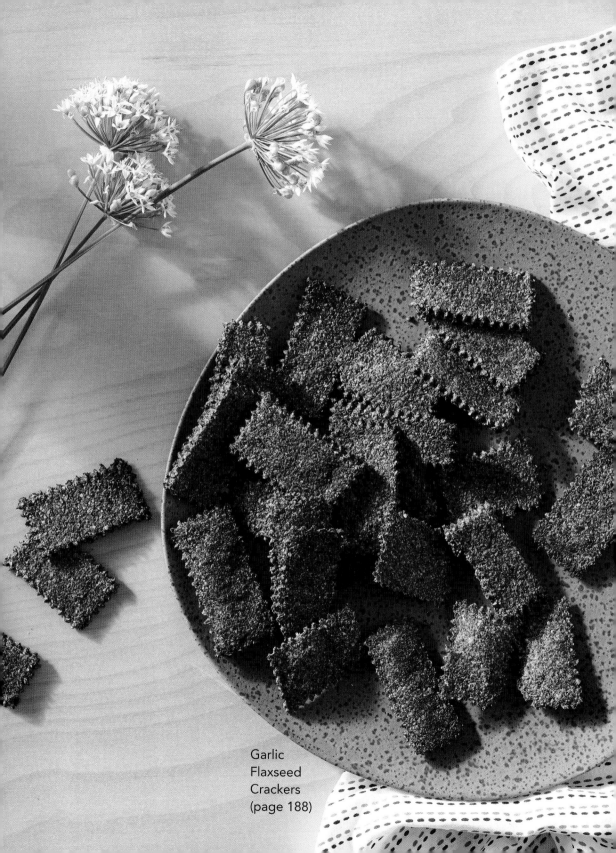

Garlic
Flaxseed
Crackers
(page 188)

ROASTED SALSA

Yield: 2 cups

*When garden vegetables are arriving in the market by the boatload,
take advantage to make this excellent salsa.*

3 tomatoes, cut in large chunks

2 Japanese or 4 small eggplants, trimmed and cut in thick slices (optional)

2 teaspoons ground cumin, divided

½ teaspoon salt, divided

¼ teaspoon black pepper, divided

2 garlic cloves, peeled and minced

2 tablespoons chopped fresh parsley

1 tablespoon chopped fresh chives

1 tablespoon chopped fresh cilantro

1 tablespoon lime juice

2 tablespoons olive oil

1 Preheat the broiler to high. Meanwhile, lightly spray 2 rimmed baking sheets with olive oil cooking spray.

2 Place the tomatoes and eggplants (optional) in a single layer on one baking sheet.

3 Sprinkle the tomatoes and eggplants with the cumin, salt, and pepper.

4 Broil for 5 to 6 minutes or until browned. Remove from the oven and set aside to cool completely.

5 Meanwhile, stir together the garlic, parsley, chives, cilantro, lime juice, and oil in a small mixing bowl.

6 When the eggplant slices are cool enough to handle, chop and add to the garlic mixture, tossing to blend.

7 Cover and refrigerate at least 30 minutes before serving.

Serving size: ¼ cup

calories	fat	protein	carbs	fiber
42.4	3.6g	0.61g	2.56g	0.7g

WALNUT & RED PEPPER SPREAD

Yield: 2 ¼ cups

This spread has just enough sweet to balance the spice.
It can be made ahead of time and refrigerated up to 3 days.

1 (12-ounce) jar roasted red bell peppers, drained

3 garlic cloves, peeled

1 cup walnuts, coarsely chopped

2 tablespoons plain, chive, or jalapeño cream cheese

2 tablespoons olive oil

1 tablespoon lemon juice

2 to 4 drops liquid stevia

1 teaspoon ground cumin

¼ teaspoon cayenne

¼ teaspoon black pepper

⅛ teaspoon onion salt

1 Place the peppers, garlic, walnuts, cream cheese, oil, lemon juice, stevia, cumin, cayenne, pepper, and salt in the bowl of a food processor.

2 Process until smooth and transfer to a serving dish. Serve immediately or refrigerate for later use.

Serving size: ¼ cup

calories	fat	protein	carbs	fiber
135	12.9g	2.4g	4.51g	1.01g

HERBED GOAT CHEESE

Yield: 1¼ cups

After one taste, you might wish you had doubled this recipe. It is terrific spread over avocado slices for breakfast or on Herbed Focaccia (page 198) for a snack.

1 (4-ounce) package plain, soft goat cheese, softened

⅔ cup small-curd cottage cheese

2 garlic cloves, peeled

2 tablespoons chopped fresh chives

2 tablespoons chopped fresh parsley

1 tablespoon chopped fresh basil

¼ teaspoon black pepper

1 Place the goat cheese, cottage cheese, garlic, chives, parsley, basil, and pepper in the bowl of a food processor. Process until smooth.

2 Cover and refrigerate at least 30 minutes before serving.

NOTE: If you want to use this as a dip, add 2 tablespoons of unsweetened almond milk to the food processor.

Serving size: ¼ cup

	calories	fat	protein	carbs	fiber
	115	8.1g	8.4g	1.67g	0.14g

CUCUMBER MINT DIP

Yield: 2 ¾ cups

*Nothing could be more refreshing on a hot afternoon that this creamy dip.
Make it and refrigerate for a cool-down snack with sliced cucumber,
celery stalks, or to accompany kabobs.*

1 cup sour cream

1 ¼ cups cream cheese

1 cup cucumber, finely
peeled, seeded, and
chopped

⅓ cup chopped fresh
mint

2 teaspoons
lemon juice

1 teaspoon finely
grated lemon zest

¼ teaspoon
white pepper

⅛ teaspoon salt

1 In a medium bowl, stir together the sour
cream, cucumber, mint, lemon juice, lemon
zest, pepper, and salt.

2 Cover and refrigerate at least 30 minutes
before serving.

Serving size: ¼ cup

calories	fat	protein	carbs	fiber
136	13.2g	2.2g	2.9g	0.16g

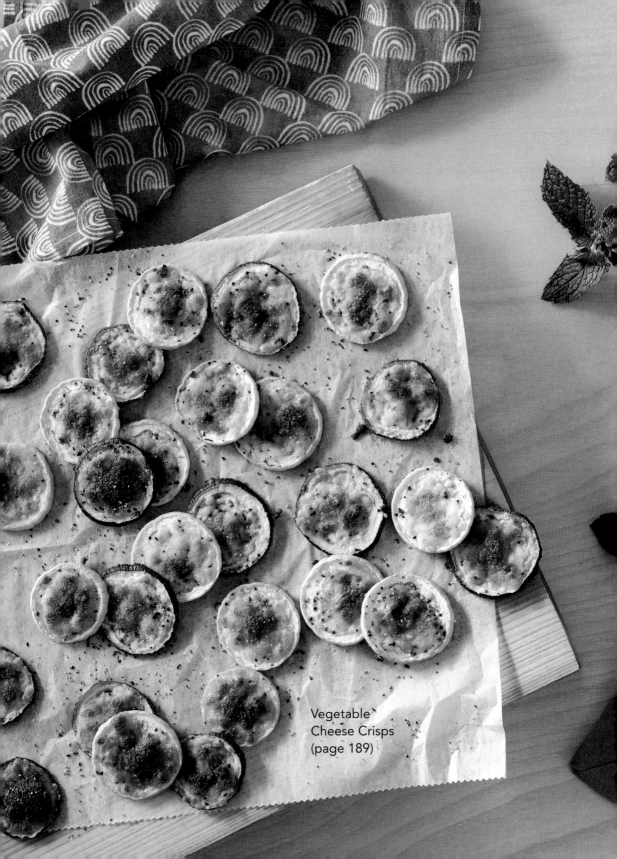

Vegetable
Cheese Crisps
(page 189)

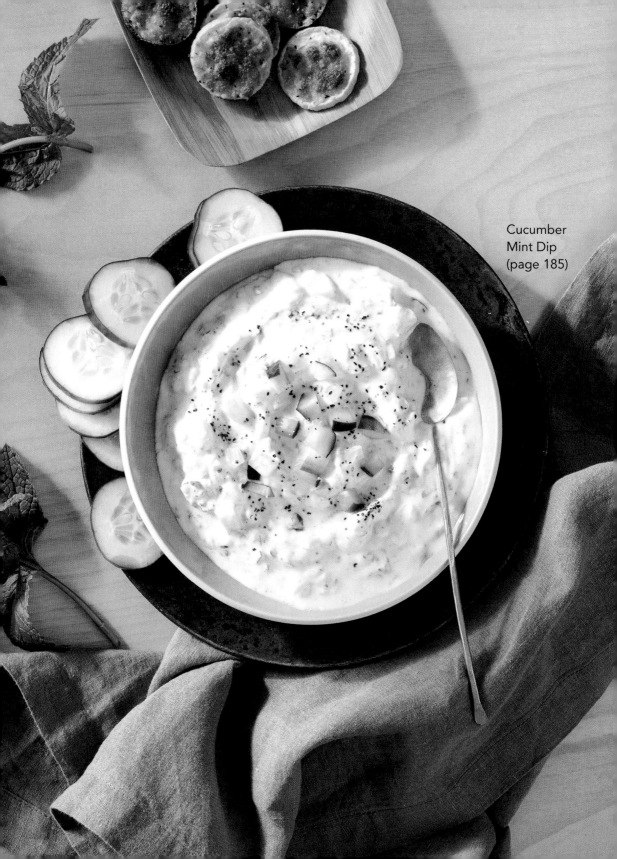

Cucumber
Mint Dip
(page 185)

GARLIC FLAXSEED CRACKERS

Yield: 8 to 10 crackers

*These richly dark crackers provide a perfect snack when
you need a bit of crunch. Cool completely on a wire rack
and if they must be stored, make sure the container is airtight.*

1½ cups
  ground flaxseed

½ teaspoon
  garlic powder

½ teaspoon
  garlic salt

½ teaspoon
  black pepper

½ cup water

1 Preheat the oven to 350 degrees. Line a baking sheet with parchment paper and set aside.

2 In a medium mixing bowl, stir together the flaxseed, garlic powder, salt, and pepper.

3 Make a well in the center of the flour mixture and add the water, stirring to form a dough.

4 Transfer the dough to a pastry cloth and roll it very thin (1⁄16 inch thick).

5 With a sharp knife or a pastry wheel, cut the dough into triangles or rectangles.

6 Place the triangles or rectangles on the prepared baking sheet, making sure they are half an inch apart.

7 Reroll and cut scraps to use all the dough.

8 Bake 25 to 30 minutes or until dry. Cool completely on a wire rack.

Serving size: 1 cracker

calories	fat	protein	carbs	fiber
113	8.9g	3.9g	6.3g	5.8g

VEGETABLE CHEESE CRISPS

Yield: 4 servings

*These crispy chips will pair well with nearly any dip or spread.
As the fresh vegetable season progresses, you can change
the produce to fit what is in abundance.*

4 zucchini, yellow straightneck squash, or Japanese eggplant, trimmed and cut in ¼-inch slices

½ teaspoon garlic salt

¼ teaspoon black pepper

1 cup grated Romano cheese

1 Preheat the oven to 425 degrees and line a baking sheet with parchment paper.

2 Place the vegetable slices on the parchment paper and sprinkle evenly with the salt and pepper.

3 Cover each slice with Romano cheese and bake 15 to 18 minutes or until golden brown. Serve warm.

calories	fat	protein	carbs	fiber
336	21g	27g	11.3g	2.8g

PARMESAN CHIPS

Yield: 12 chips

*Crisp and crunchy, these cheese chips are super easy to make.
Store any leftovers in an airtight container.*

½ heaping cup
shredded Parmesan
cheese

1 teaspoon
dried parsley*

¼ teaspoon
black pepper

1 Preheat the oven to 400 degrees and line a baking sheet with parchment paper.

2 Using a tablespoon, place Parmesan cheese in mounds a couple of inches apart on a baking sheet and spread each into 2-inch rounds, making about 12 rounds.

3 Sprinkle the tops evenly with the parsley and pepper.

4 Bake 7 to 8 minutes or until golden brown.

5 Remove from the oven and lift the parchment paper onto a large cooling rack. Allow the chips to cool completely, and then remove them with a thin spatula.

*NOTE: For a bit of spice, you can substitute ¼ teaspoon cayenne for the parsley, or just sprinkle ¼ teaspoon cayenne in addition to the parsley.

Serving size: 4 chips

calories	fat	protein	carbs	fiber
60	3.7g	5.3g	1.5g	0.2g

CHEDDAR CHIPS

Yield: 20 chips

This is a variation of Parmesan Chips that is made the same, but with a different flavor. Use sharp or extra-sharp Cheddar for the most noticeable cheese taste. These will have a bit of grease on top after baked, so take a paper towel and gently dab the tops after baking.

1 cup shredded sharp or extra sharp Cheddar cheese

1 teaspoon garlic powder

¼ teaspoon salt

¼ teaspoon paprika

1 Preheat the oven to 400 degrees and line a baking sheet with parchment paper.

2 Using a tablespoon, place Cheddar cheese in mounds a couple of inches apart on a baking sheet and spread each into 2-inch rounds.

3 Sprinkle the tops evenly with the garlic powder, salt, and paprika.

4 Bake 6 to 7 minutes or until golden brown.

5 Remove from the oven and lift the parchment paper onto a large cooling rack. Allow the chips to cool completely then remove them with a thin spatula.

Serving size: 4 chips

calories	fat	protein	carbs	fiber
94	7.5g	5.3g	1.2g	0g

SUMMER SQUASH "CHIPS"

Yield: 3 servings

*This uses a culinary trick that caterers have been doing for years.
It will crisp up the vegetables beautifully.*

2 zucchini, trimmed and cut in ¼-inch slices

2 yellow straightneck squash, trimmed and cut in ¼-inch slices

¼ teaspoon salt

1 Place the zucchini and squash slices in a large bowl.

2 Cover with ice and refrigerate 30 minutes.

3 Drain and pat dry with paper towels.

4 Sprinkle with the salt and serve with your favorite dip.

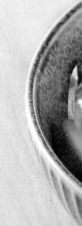

calories	fat	protein	carbs	fiber
43	0.7g	3.1g	8.4g	2.7g

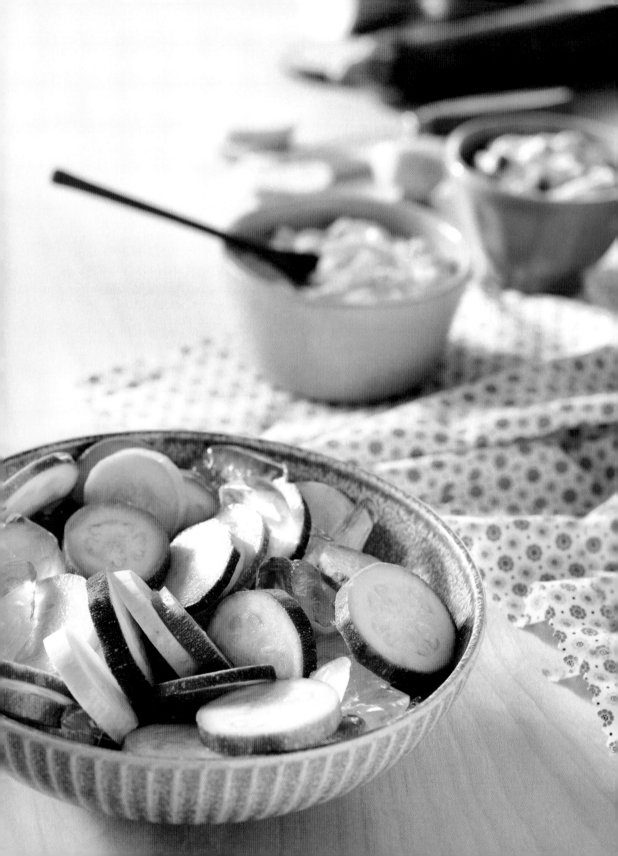

LOADED RADISHES

Yields: 4 servings

Missing potatoes but want to stay in the Keto Zone? Look no further than this winning dish. You may never crave a loaded baked potato again.

2 tablespoons avocado oil

1 pound radishes, quartered

1 teaspoon minced garlic

½ teaspoon salt

½ teaspoon ground black pepper

¼ cups grated Cheddar cheese

4 slices nitrate free bacon, cooked and crumbled

1 tablespoon green onions, chopped

4 tablespoons sour cream (optional)

1 Heat the oil in a large skillet over medium heat.

2 Add the radishes to the skillet and top with garlic powder, salt, and pepper. Cook for 10 to 15 minutes, stirring occasionally until the radishes have softened and browned.

3 Turn off heat and top radishes with cheese and bacon. Cover the pan and let sit for 2 to 4 minutes or until cheese has melted.

4 Sprinkle with green onions and serve warm.

*OPTION: top with 2 tablespoons of sour cream per serving.

calories	fat	protein	carbs	fiber
188	15.8g	6.7g	5.3g	1.9g

BELL PEPPER NACHOS

Yields: 2 servings

*Looking for a snack that will tide you over until dinner?
Or do you have a late night ahead of you and you need something
filling to keep your energy up? These nachos are sure to satisfy!*

½ pound grass-fed ground beef

2 green bell peppers

2 tablespoons avocado oil

¼ teaspoon chili powder

¼ teaspoon ground cumin

¼ teaspoon garlic powder

½ teaspoon salt

½ teaspoon black pepper

Pinch of red pepper flakes (optional)

½ cup shredded Mexican blend cheese

1   Preheat oven to 400 degrees.

2   Cut the bell peppers through the stem into six equal pieces, removing the stem, seeds, and membrane.

3   Place the peppers cut side up spread evenly on a small baking sheet. Drizzle with 1 tablespoon of oil.

4   Heat 1 tablespoon oil in a medium skillet over medium-high heat. Add beef, chili powder, ground cumin, garlic powder, salt, pepper, and crushed red pepper (optional). Cook until beef is cooked through and browned, about 7 to 10 minutes. Break up the beef as it cooks.

5   Spoon ground beef into the prepared peppers. Divide cheese between peppers.

6   Bake until cheese melts and peppers begin to soften, about 7 minutes.

7   Remove from oven and add desired toppings. Serve warm.

TOPPINGS: Top with a small scoop of the Addictive Guacamole (page 176), the Roasted Salsa (page 182), or a dollop of sour cream.

calories	fat	protein	carbs	fiber
589	44.4g	38.4g	9g	1.7g

DEVILED EGGS

Yield: 4 servings

Whether you use these as a snack, side dish, or breakfast, the basic preparation is the same. You can vary the toppings any way you want!

4 eggs

4 tablespoons
avocado mayonnaise

1 tablespoon chopped
sweet pickle

¼ teaspoon salt

¼ teaspoon
black pepper

1 Place the eggs in a medium saucepan and add enough cold water to cover by 1 inch.

2 Place over medium-high heat. As soon as the water comes to a boil, remove the pan from the heat and cover. Let stand 15 minutes.

3 Drain and transfer the eggs to a bowl of ice water. Let them stand until cool.

4 Peel the eggs and cut in half lengthwise. Transfer the yolks to a bowl and mash with a fork.

5 Stir in the mayonnaise, pickle, salt, and pepper.

6 Place the egg whites on a serving plate and spoon the yolk mixture into each egg.

7 Cover and refrigerate at least 20 minutes. Serve chilled.

GARNISHES: Top each egg half with a small salad shrimp, sliced olives, chopped herbs, a sprinkling of paprika, or minced peppers.

calories	fat	protein	carbs	fiber
84	6g	6.3g	0.7g	0g

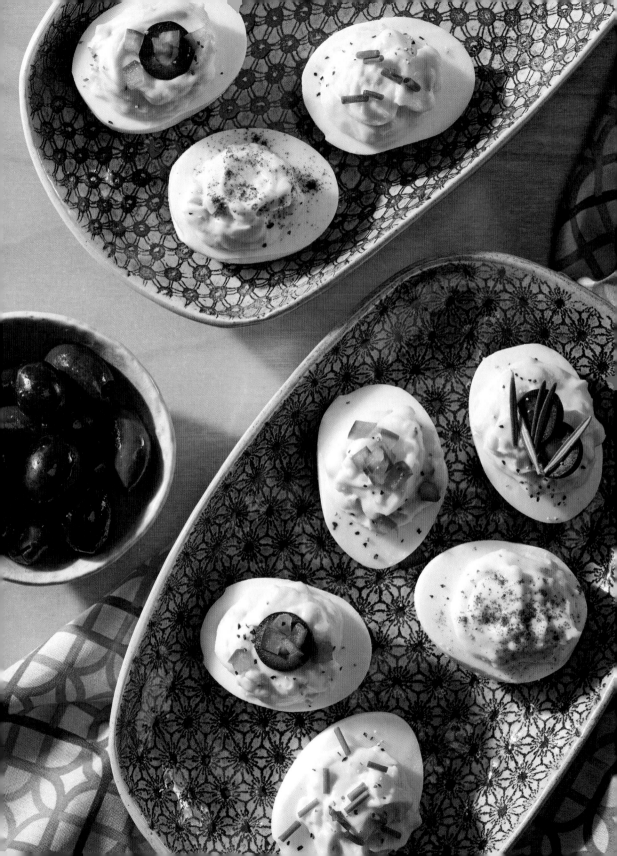

DILL PICKLES

Yield: 6 pints

Summer is the time of year for pickle making. That's when cucumbers flood the market, and you can easily find plenty identical in size.

3 cups white vinegar

3 cups water

6 tablespoons pickling salt

12 sprigs fresh dill

6 garlic cloves, peeled

3 teaspoons mustard seeds, divided

30 cucumbers (4 inches long), trimmed

6 canning jars

1 In a medium saucepan, bring the vinegar, water, and salt to a boil over medium-high heat to make a brine solution.

2 Meanwhile place 1 sprig of dill, 1 garlic clove, and ½ teaspoon of the mustard seeds in the bottom of each pint canning jar. Pack the cucumbers into six canning jars that have been washed and sterilized.

3 When jars are half filled with cucumbers, add 1 more dill sprig and complete packing with cucumbers.

4 Fill with the brine solution and leave ½-inch headspace. Remove any air bubbles, wipe the jar rims, and screw on the lids.

5 Process 10 minutes in a boiling water bath.

6 Place on a wire rack away from drafts to cool completely. Store at room temperature.

Serving size: 1 pickle

calories	fat	protein	carbs	fiber
29	0.2g	1.1g	5.7g	0.8g

NO BAKE TRAIL MIX

Yield: 3 ¼ cups

*Feel free to increase or decrease the ingredient amounts listed
to fit your own taste.*

1 cup macadamias

½ cup unsweetened
coconut flakes

½ cup dark chocolate
(85% cocoa or
higher), coarsely
chopped

½ cup pecan halves

½ cup walnut halves

¼ cup sliced almonds

1   Place the macadamias, coconut, chocolate,
pecans, walnuts, and almonds in a large
zip-top bag.

2   Seal and shake to mix.

3   Store in the refrigerator.

calories	fat	protein	carbs	fiber
138	12.5g	2.5g	5.6g	2.1g

HERBED FOCACCIA

Yield: 12 servings

Flatbreads like focaccia are great for dipping in flavored oils or accompanying soups and salads. It can also be sliced and frozen. Make sure the flaxseed is coarsely ground rather than finely ground to give the bread some texture.

2 cups coarsely ground flaxseed or sunflower seeds

1 tablespoon baking powder

1 teaspoon dried basil

1 teaspoon dried oregano

1 teaspoon dried parsley or chives

1 teaspoon garlic salt

⅛ teaspoon black pepper

5 eggs

½ cup water

⅓ cup avocado oil

1 Preheat the oven to 350 degrees and line a 13x9-inch baking sheet with parchment paper, making sure it extends over the sides. Very lightly grease the bottom with olive oil cooking spray and set aside.

2 Stir together the flaxseed or sunflower seeds, baking powder, basil, oregano, parsley or chives, salt, and pepper in a large mixing bowl. Set aside.

3 Place the eggs, water, and oil in a blender and blend for 15 to 20 seconds.

4 Add the egg mixture to the flaxseed or sunflower mixture and stir to blend.

5 Let stand for 3 minutes before spreading evenly in the prepared pan.

6 Bake for 20 minutes or until golden brown.

7 Using the parchment paper, lift the bread out of the pan and remove the parchment paper. Place on a wire rack to cool completely before slicing and serving.

calories	fat	protein	carbs	fiber
184	16g	6.1g	6g	5.2g

SEED BREAD

Yield: 12 servings

*You'll need some time for making this bread so don't get in a hurry.
It is the same process to line the pan as it is for the Herbed Focaccia,
so make sure you have enough overhang of the parchment paper
to use as a handle for lifting the bread from the pan.*

1 cup ground
  hemp seeds

¾ cup ground
  pumpkin seeds

¾ cup ground
  flaxseed

¾ cup raw
  sunflower seeds

3 tablespoons
  ground chia seeds

3 tablespoons
  sesame seeds

1 teaspoon
  seasoned salt

½ teaspoon powdered
  stevia

1½ cups water

1 tablespoon +
  1½ teaspoons
  coconut oil, melted

1 tablespoon +
  1½ teaspoons ghee,
  melted

1 In a large mixing bowl, stir together the hemp seeds, pumpkin seeds, flaxseed, sunflower seeds, chia seeds, sesame seeds, salt, and stevia.

2 Combine the water, coconut oil, and ghee in a quart jar with a tight-fitting lid.

3 Shake to emulsify and add to the seed mixture. Stir well, and let stand at room temperature 2½ hours. It will have a batter-like consistency.

4 Preheat the oven to 350 degrees and line a loaf pan with parchment paper, allowing the paper to hang off the ends.

5 Transfer the batter to the prepared pan and bake 20 minutes.

6 Rotate the pan and bake an additional 50 minutes.

7 Cool in the pan 5 minutes, then using the parchment paper as a handle, remove the bread from the pan.

8 Peel off the paper and cool completely on a wire rack before slicing and serving.

calories	fat	protein	carbs	fiber
424	37g	19g	11.7g	6.9g

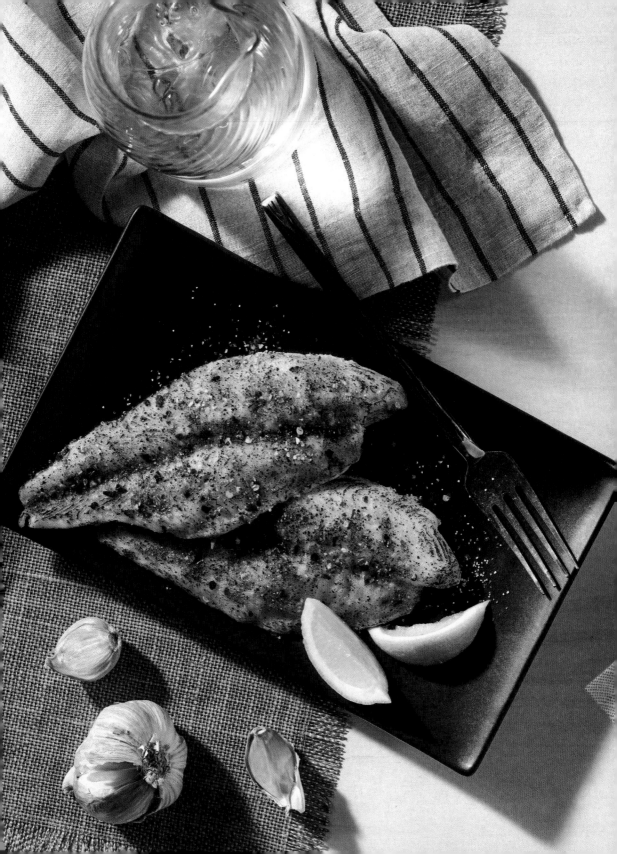

APPENDICES

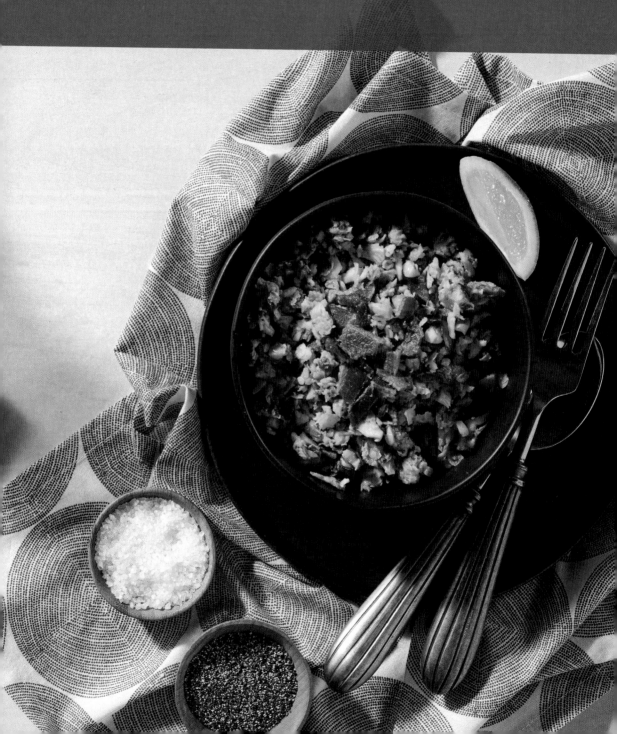

APPENDIX A

Depending on your health and your sickness, one or more of these supplements and Keto Zone products may help speed you along the trail toward health. You can order your Divine Health Nutritional Products by calling (407) 732-6952 or visiting Shop.DrColbert.com.

SUPPLEMENTS

- Green Supremefood: a whole food nutritional powder with fermented grasses and vegetables
- Red Supremefood: a whole food nutritional powder with antiaging fruits
- Enhanced multivitamin
- Living probiotic
- Living chia with probiotics

KETO ZONE PRODUCTS

Instant Ketones contain Betahydroxybuturate (BHB), a key ingredient that speeds up the process of entering ketosis. It typically takes 2 days to 2 weeks to enter ketosis, but Instant Ketones can help you enter ketosis almost immediately. A coconut flavor hides the salty flavor that comes with BHB. Start by taking ½ scoop in water or a smoothie and gradually increase to a full scoop per day.

Hydrolyzed Collagen is comprised of chicken collagen, partly containing Type I collagen but primarily containing Type II collagen. As you age, your body slowly loses collagen, which is found throughout the body, including hair, nails, joints, bones, heart, and skin. The most common form of joint pain is caused from the deterioration of collagen in the cartilage of the joints, and Type II collagen helps support connective tissue. Your body's joints and skin repair themselves at night, so it's best to take ½ to 1 scoop in any liquid 30 minutes before bedtime. New chocolate flavor is now available.

MCT Oil Powder is made of healthy fats that help support a healthy heart and brain. Every cell of your body depends on lipids or fats to survive. In fact, your brain contains over 60 percent fats. MCT Oil also helps the liver produce ketone bodies, which put the body into ketosis and set the body up to burn fat. Take 1 scoop of MCT oil Powder in a cup of coffee in the morning as an alternative creamer, or mix into any hot liquid to avoid clumping. Flavors include coconut, hazelnut, and French vanilla.

ICED Krill contains essential fats such as DHA and EPA, which provide the brain with cognitive fuel. This formula also contains naturally occurring astaxanthin, one of the most powerful natural antioxidants found, which helps support healthy eyes while also neutralizing harmful free radicals. Krill are small crustaceans that are caught off the coast of Antarctica. They are then immediately ICED and processed onboard the shipping vessel to ensure optimal quality. ICED Krill is then encapsulated in a special nitrogen flush process that maintains its freshness, and, because of a special double-banded process, the krill is completely odorless.

Fat-Zyme is a digestive enzyme designed to break down fats and vegetables. The Keto Zone diet is a diet high in healthy fats and vegetables, and since our bodies do not naturally produce large amounts of lipase, which breaks down fats, Fat-Zyme fills this void.

APPENDIX B

HEALTHY CARBS FOR FINDING YOUR KCL

After you have reached your ideal weight, it is time to slowly increase your daily carb intake from the Keto Zone's starting point of 20 grams per day. At the start of each week, increase your daily carb intake by a total of 10 grams. After a week at 30 grams of carbs per day, increase to 40 grams for the next week, and so on. When you get to the point where you are neither gaining nor losing weight, you are at your KCL, your Keto Carb Limit.

These healthy carbs are great to use as you increase your carb intake in 10-gram increments:

- Beans, cooked (kidney, lima, navy, pinto, white, lentils, or brown): ¼ cup, 10 g. carbs
- Peas: raw ½ cup, 10 g. carbs
- Hummus: 4 Tbsp., 10 g. carbs
- Seeds:
  - ¤ Chia seeds: 3 Tbsp., 12 g. carbs
  - ¤ Flaxseed: 3 Tbsp., 9 g. carbs
  - ¤ Pumpkin seeds: ½ cup, 15 g. carbs
  - ¤ Sunflower seeds: ¼ cup, 7 g. carbs
- Nuts, dry or roasted:
  - ¤ Almonds: ½ cup, 13 g. carbs
  - ¤ Cashews: ¼ cup, 10 g. carbs
  - ¤ Peanuts: ¼ cup, 7.5 g. carbs
  - ¤ Pecans: ½ cup, 7 g. carbs
- Cream cheese (regular): 8 oz., 9 g. carbs
- Full-fat yogurt: 8 oz., 10 g. carbs
- Low glycemic fruits
  - ¤ Apples: ½ medium apple, 9 g. carbs
  - ¤ Blueberries: ½ cup, 10 g. carbs
  - ¤ Raspberries: ½ cup, 9 g. carbs
  - ¤ Strawberries: 1 cup, 12 g. carbs

APPENDIX C
COOKING EQUIVALENTS CHART

Amount	Equals	
16 dashes	1 teaspoon	
8 pinches	1 teaspoon	
3 teaspoons	1 tablespoon	½ fl. oz.
⅛ cup	2 tablespoons	1 fl. oz.
¼ cup	4 tablespoons	2 fl. oz.
⅓ cup	5 tablespoons + 1 teaspoon	2 ⅔ fl. oz.
½ cup	8 tablespoons	4 fl. oz.
⅔ cup	10 tablespoons + 2 teaspoons	5 ⅓ fl. oz.
¾ cup	12 tablespoons	6 fl. oz.
1 cup	16 tablespoons	8 fl. oz.
1 pint	2 cups	16 fl. oz.
1 quart	4 cups	2 pints
1 gallon	16 cups	4 quarts

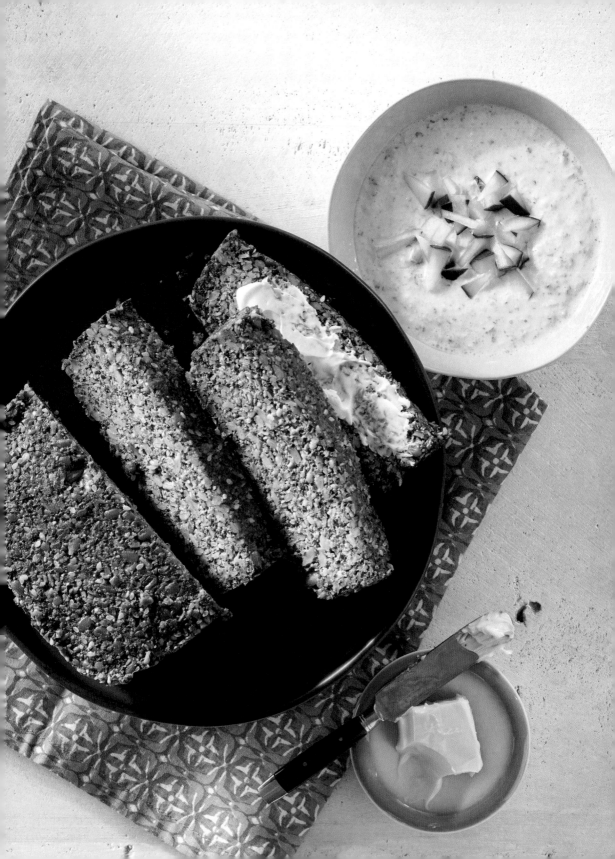

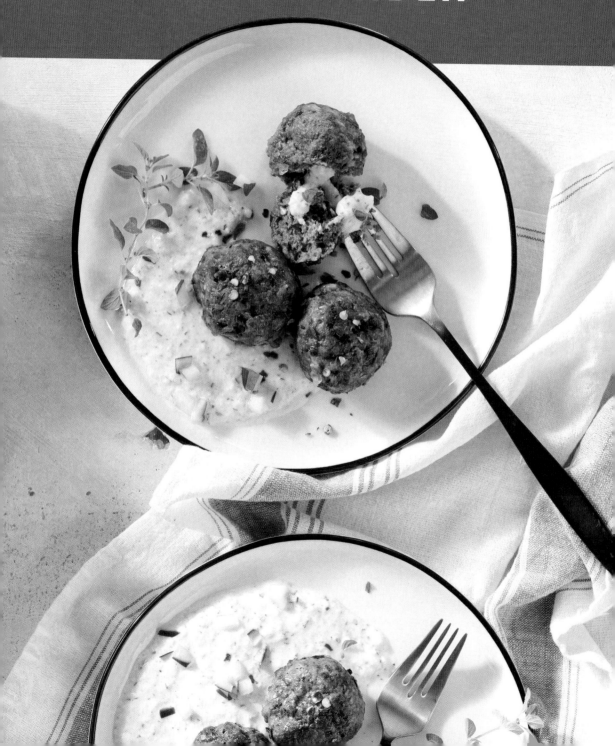

RECIPE INDEX

BASICS

BREAKFAST

LUNCH

DINNER

GENERAL INDEX

A

alcohol 20

almonds 31, 69, 72, 76, 90, 159, 163, 169, 199, 206

  almond butter 77, 160, 166, 169, 172

  almond extract 72, 76, 158

  almond flour 72, 73, 148

  almond milk 56, 63, 65, 66, 68, 72, 76, 77, 78, 87, 168, 184

  almond oil 41, 72, 90

amino acid 13, 14, 33

anchovy fillets 51

appetite 4, 7, 8, 12, 14, 19

apple cider vinegar 23 (*see also* cider vinegar)

apples 206

artichoke hearts 148, 177

artificial sweeteners 19, 20

arugula 96, 124

asparagus spears 86, 113

avocado 46, 59, 84, 128, 152, 162, 176, 184

  avocado mayonnaise 41, 48, 49, 69, 90, 98, 110, 111, 121, 130, 179, 196

  avocado oil 24, 26, 27, 30, 46, 48, 49, 59, 65, 66, 68, 77, 78, 82, 84, 86, 88, 99, 100, 102, 106, 107, 110, 112, 120, 122, 131, 132, 140, 152, 154, 176, 194, 195, 200

B

bacon 14, 59, 147, 178, 194

baking powder 72, 73, 170, 200

baking soda 72

balsamic vinegar 153

basil 26, 46, 86, 94, 116, 126, 127, 130, 135, 153, 184, 200

bay leaf 38, 39, 86

beans 19, 206

beef 87, 103, 104, 195

  bones 38

  brisket 138

  filet mignon 136

  rump roast 135

  sirloin steak 139

  stock 135

bell pepper

  green 139, 179, 195

  red 83

beverages 6, 14, 20, 25

  black tea 20, 33

  coffee 20, 27, 29, 31, 33

  fruit juice 20

  green tea 20, 33

  water 9, 32

  beverages (list) 25

blackberries 77

black olives 92

black pepper (*required in most recipes*)

blood pressure 15

blueberries 77, 206

bocconcini 153

bok choy 68, 95, 102

bone broth 38, 84, 135, 154

BPA 19, 40

broccoli 14, 68, 113, 120

  rabe 142

  spears 113

Brussels sprouts 68, 113, 147

butter, grass-fed 12, 19, 24, 26, 27, 28, 30, 42, 54, 55, 56, 59, 62, 63, 64, 69, 72, 74, 86, 88, 95, 96, 99, 102, 107, 108, 110, 111, 112, 116, 117, 118, 120, 122, 123, 124, 126, 128, 134, 135, 136, 146, 164, 167

C

cacao nibs 162

calories 12, 27, 28, 30

  caloric intake 10

cancer 1, 14, 17, 19

canned food 19

capers 46, 51

carbohydrate 6, 7, 8, 9, 11, 13, 14, 18

  carb intake 7, 9, 12, 13, 14, 18, 20, 27, 31, 206

  carb sensitivity 9

cardamom 159

cashews 22, 23, 206

cauliflower 68, 82, 99, 113, 150

lettuce (*con't*)
  romaine 91, 107
  salad greens 46
lime 92, 128
  juice 41, 48, 92, 103, 128, 130, 152, 164, 173, 176, 182
  zest 107, 128, 173
liquid aminos 41, 44, 48, 95, 102, 103, 107
lose weight 1, 3, 4, 7, 8, 11, 12, 15, 17, 27, 33, 206, 217
low-carb 1, 25, 33
low-fat 7, 9, 11, 13, 19, 32

M

macadamia nuts 173, 199
MCT oil 24, 27, 28, 30, 205
  MCT oil powder 24, 27, 28, 54, 77, 166, 172, 205
meat (list) 22
medicine 5
mental illness 1
metabolism 7, 14, 28
mint 185
mint extract 162
monk fruit 6, 19
monounsaturated fats 7, 10, (list) 24, 28
multivitamin 25, 204
mushrooms 56, 73, 96, 148
  button mushrooms 139
mustard seed 198

N

nut butter 7

nutmeg 84
nuts (list) 22

O

obesity 1, 19
oils 24
olive oil, extra-virgin 23, 24, 26, 30, 31, 32, 45, 50, 51, 57, 58, 65, 69, 72, 73, 76, 87, 88, 91, 92, 94, 95, 96, 102, 103, 104, 107, 110, 116, 117, 118, 123, 124, 127, 142, 143, 152, 153, 182, 183
olives 196
  pimiento-stuffed olives 91
omega-3 10, 13, 25
onion 38, 39, 56, 59, 84, 86, 100, 103, 105, 135, 177
onion powder 144
onion salt 41, 44, 50, 66, 73, 88, 91, 108, 120, 121, 131, 135, 140, 142, 148, 150, 177, 179, 183
orange 20, 64, 158
oregano 50, 91, 96, 105, 126, 132, 135, 143, 200

P

pancetta 147
paper cups 160
paprika 44, 69, 73, 87, 92, 110, 120, 121, 131, 140, 144, 177, 191, 196
parsley 49, 51, 62, 63, 64, 68, 73, 86, 99, 105, 126, 132, 143, 178, 182, 184, 190, 200

peanuts 23, 31, 206
  peanut butter 77, 78
pecan 169, 199
  butter 160
peppercorns 38, 39
pepper (*see* black pepper, red pepper, or white pepper)
peppers 196
pickle 196
pickling salt 198
pine nuts 124
polyunsaturated fats 7, 10, 30
pork
  bones 38
  loin 143
  loin chops 142
  pork tenderloins 140
  shoulder 144
poultry (list) 21
probiotic 204
processed food 3, 19
  meat 14
prosciutto 124, 132
protein 1, 7, 9, 10, 11, 13, 14, 18, 20, 21, 22, 25, 27, 28, 29, 30, 77, 78, 87
proteins 21
pumpkin pie spice 74
pumpkin purée 74
  seeds 159, 201

R

radicchio 91
radish 194
raspberries 72, 77, 206
raw veggies (list) 23
red onion 111
red pepper 105, 118, 122, 132, 142, 147, 176, 195

rosemary 38, 68, 112, 134, 140, 143

S

sage 134

salmon 70, 98, 117, 118, 122, 123

salt 31, (*required in most recipes*)

saturated fat 7, 10, (list) 24

sauces 6, 20

scallions 110

scallops 96, 124

sea salt 31, 169, 172

seasoned salt 201

sesame seeds 87, 95, 106, 201

shallot 66, 82, 90, 94, 99, 102, 154, 176

shellfish (list) 21

shrimp 83, 91, 96, 179, 196

sleep disorders 4

snow peas 113

sour cream 45, 48, 69, 83, 104, 110, 130, 150, 170, 177, 185, 194, 195

spices (list) 26

spinach 59, 65, 66, 73, 92, 122, 154, 177

squash 113, 192, 212

straightneck 189, 192

starches 6, 9, 11, 20, 29

stevia 6, 19, 20, 28, 29, 41, 54, 72, 76, 144, 159, 160, 162, 163, 164, 166, 167, 170, 183, 201

liquid stevia 41, 72, 74, 77, 78, 159, 160, 163, 170, 172, 173, 183

strawberry 72, 77, 206

sugar 3, 6, 9, 11, 13, 14, 15, 19, 20, 27, 29, 31

sugar snap 113

sunflower seeds 173, 200, 201

supplements 5, (list) 25, 204

sweets 6

syrup 72

T

tahini 48

tarragon vinegar 123

thyme 38, 39, 112, 120, 126, 130, 134, 143

tilapia 102, 116, 121

tomato 26, 44, 56, 59, 66, 92, 94, 99, 148, 182

cherry 98

grape 153

Roma 94

turkey 134

ground 69, 100

tenderloins 103, 106

sausage 56, 59, 100

bacon 59

turmeric 86

type 2 diabetes 1, 4, 17, 18

U

unhealthy oils 19

urine test strip 11

V

vanilla extract 163, 168

vegetables 23

W

walnuts 96, 169, 183, 199

weight loss 15, 17, (*see also* lose weight)

wheat 19

white pepper 42, 45, 46, 48, 49, 68, 83, 99, 104, 123, 138, 148, 176, 185

white vinegar 198

Z

zucchini 84, 86, 88, 94, 103, 189, 192

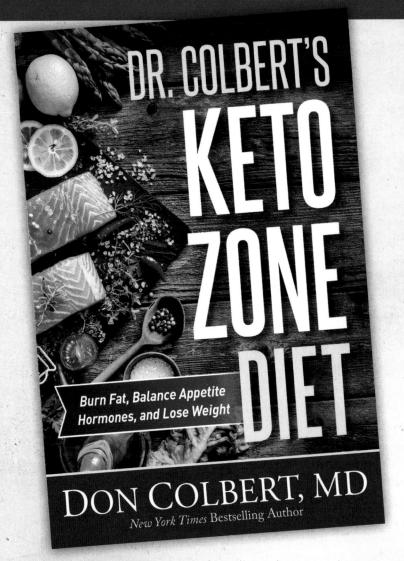